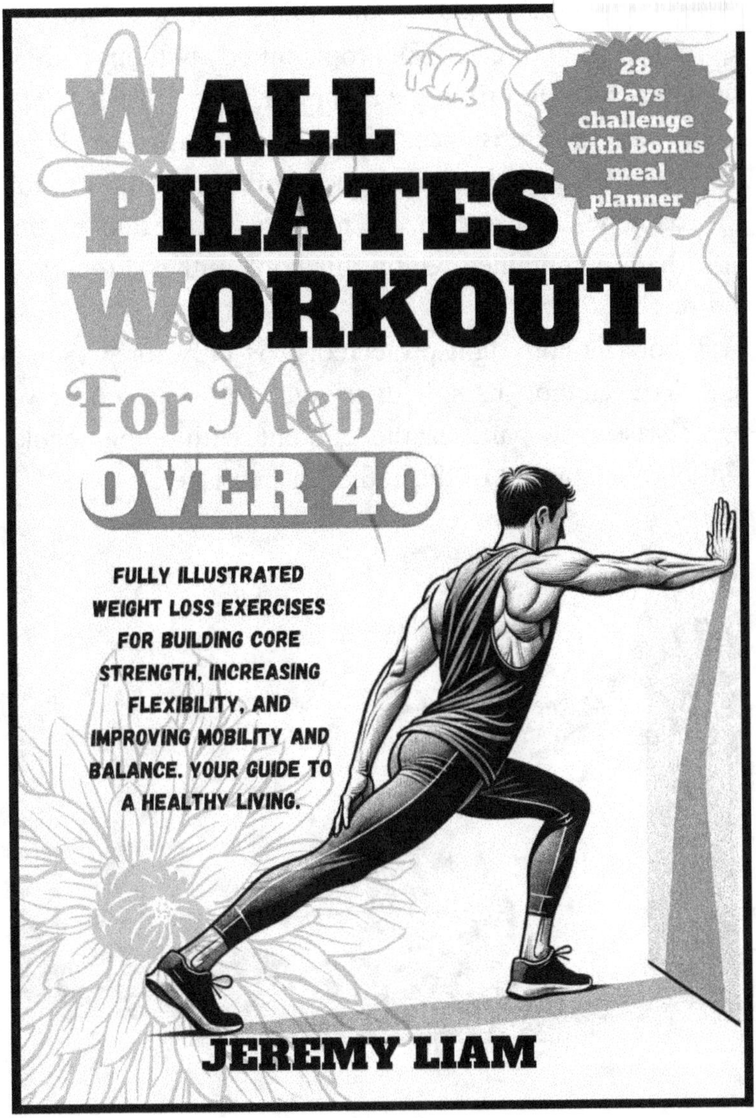

WALL PILATES WORKOUT

For Men

OVER 40

28 Days challenge with Bonus meal planner

FULLY ILLUSTRATED WEIGHT LOSS EXERCISES FOR BUILDING CORE STRENGTH, INCREASING FLEXIBILITY, AND IMPROVING MOBILITY AND BALANCE. YOUR GUIDE TO A HEALTHY LIVING.

JEREMY LIAM

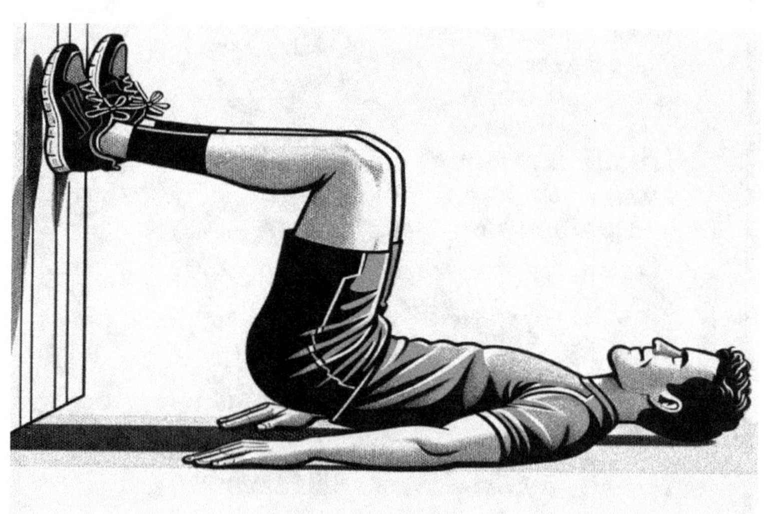

TABLE OF CONTENTS

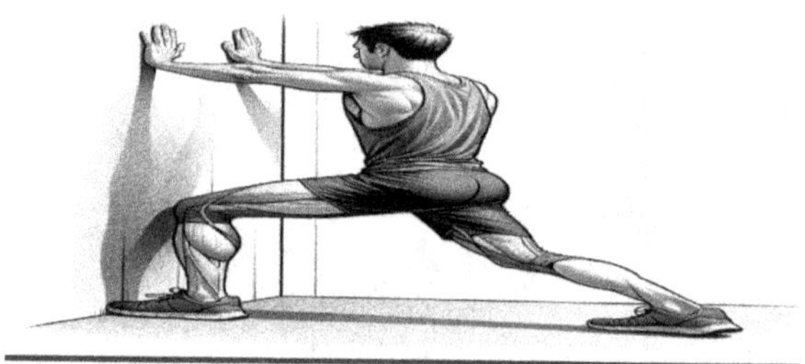

INTRODUCTION

I first met John in a typical, bustling office environment, where the glow of screens was as constant as the ticking of the clock. He was an office worker, dedicated and hardworking, but visibly struggling with his health. John was overweight, and the sedentary nature of his job had led to a decline in his mobility, balance, and overall physical well-being. It was clear that his constant engagement with screens and lack of physical activity had not only impacted his body but also his mental state. Every attempt at traditional exercises had been a challenge too intense, leaving him demotivated and more inclined to avoid physical activity.

When I introduced John to Wall Pilates, there was understandable skepticism. Here was a man who had been let down by the high-intensity routines that just didn't suit his body's needs. I explained to him how Wall Pilates, with its emphasis on controlled movements and lower intensity, was different. The support of the wall would offer him the stability he lacked, and the exercises were designed to gradually build strength, flexibility, and core stability – exactly what he needed.

To kickstart John's journey, we embarked on a 28-day Wall Pilates challenge. This structured plan was designed to gradually introduce him to various exercises, focusing on improving his mobility, balance, and coordination, one day at a time. The challenge provided a clear path, helping John to see tangible progress, keeping him motivated and engaged.

Day by day, John's dedication to the 28-day challenge brought remarkable changes. His mobility improved, allowing him to perform daily tasks with ease that were previously challenging. His balance and coordination saw significant improvements, reducing the risk of falls and injuries. Importantly, his core strength improved, which was pivotal in supporting his spine and overall posture – crucial for someone spending long hours at a desk.

The changes weren't just physical. John's mental health and overall outlook on life improved dramatically. He felt more energetic, his mood improved, and he developed a newfound confidence. Wall Pilates was not just an exercise routine for him; it became a gateway to a healthier lifestyle.

As the 28-day challenge concluded, John was a transformed man. He had lost weight, gained strength, and most importantly, found a routine that he could stick to without feeling overwhelmed. He continued practicing Wall Pilates, incorporating it into his daily routine, and even started advocating its benefits to his colleagues.

John's story is a testament to the transformative power of the right kind of exercise. Wall Pilates proved to be the perfect fit for someone who had been let down by traditional fitness routines. It showed that with the right approach, patience, and guidance, anyone could overcome their physical and mental barriers to lead a healthier, more fulfilling life. John's journey from a screen-bound office worker to a healthier, happier individual is a source of inspiration for anyone looking to make a change in their life.

As a seasoned gym instructor, my journey into the world of Wall Pilates has been both enlightening and transformative, not just for me but for many of the men I've had the pleasure of guiding. In the introductory chapter of this book, we delve into the fascinating origins of Pilates, exploring its evolution and particularly how Wall Pilates has emerged as a unique and powerful variant of this renowned fitness discipline.

Pilates, traditionally known for its emphasis on core strength, flexibility, and mindfulness, has often been mistakenly categorized as a workout more suited for women. However, through my years of experience in fitness training, I have witnessed first-hand the remarkable benefits it offers men, especially when adapted to the specific needs of the male body. Wall Pilates, with its focus on leveraging wall support, introduces an innovative approach that intensifies these benefits, making it an ideal practice for men of all ages and fitness levels.

In the gym, I've seen men initially approach Pilates with a degree of skepticism, only to find themselves surprised by its challenging nature and the deep, rewarding muscle work it provides. Wall Pilates, in particular, adds an element of stability and resistance that enhances traditional Pilates exercises, making them more accessible to those who are just starting while offering advanced practitioners a new level of intensity.

One of the greatest strengths of Wall Pilates is its adaptability. Whether you're a seasoned athlete looking for a workout that complements and enhances your existing regimen, or you're stepping into the gym for the first time in years, Wall Pilates offers a scalable, low-impact, yet highly effective way to improve your strength, posture, and overall well-being. Throughout this book, I'll share insights and techniques honed from my years of practice, guiding you through a journey that will not only transform your body but also your approach to fitness and health.

We will explore how Wall Pilates, with its unique blend of strength, balance, and flexibility training, addresses common issues men face in their fitness journeys, such as muscle imbalances and the risk of injury. This method offers a holistic approach to fitness that is often missing in traditional gym workouts, providing a perfect balance between strength and flexibility, power and poise.

Join me on this journey through the world of Wall Pilates, as we break down misconceptions, build up strength, and pave the way to a healthier, more balanced lifestyle. Whether you're looking to enhance your current fitness routine, recover from an injury, or simply find a new way to challenge yourself, Wall Pilates is a journey worth embarking on.

CHAPTER 1: HOW IT ALL STARTED

The origins of Pilates, much like the exercise form itself, are rooted in the principles of strength, flexibility, and mindful awareness. As a gym instructor, my journey into the depths of Pilates has been as much a discovery of its history as it has been a personal and professional evolution.

Pilates was born out of the genius of Joseph Pilates, a man whose life story is as fascinating as the method he created. Born in Germany in the late 19th century, Joseph Pilates was a sickly child, suffering from ailments like asthma and rickets. However, his determination to overcome his physical limitations led him to explore various forms of exercise, from gymnastics to boxing and even yoga. This eclectic mix of disciplines formed the foundation of what would later become Pilates.

During World War I, Pilates found himself in an internment camp in England, where he began refining his method, initially to rehabilitate fellow internees who were suffering from injuries and illnesses. Using whatever he could find, from bed springs to beer keg rings, Pilates devised equipment and exercises that emphasized control, precision, and fluid movement. This was the birth of what he called "Contrology," now known as Pilates.

The evolution of Pilates

As a gym instructor, I've always been captivated by how Pilates was ahead of its time. In an era where physical fitness was often about brute strength or endurance, Pilates emphasized the balance of body and mind, and the importance of injury prevention. His method was about the harmonious and complete coordination of body, mind, and spirit - a philosophy that resonates deeply with me both personally and professionally.

After the war, Pilates moved to the United States, where he opened his first studio in New York City, attracting a diverse crowd, from dancers and athletes to the general public. His method gained popularity, particularly in the dance community, for its ability to rebuild strength while maintaining flexibility and preventing injury.

In my years of instructing, I've seen how Pilates' principles have endured and evolved. It's not just a form of exercise; it's a path to better health and a more balanced life. The Wall Pilates we focus on now, especially suited for men over 40, is a testament to the adaptability and timelessness of Pilates' vision. It provides a perfect blend of strength, control, and mindfulness, tailored to the needs of an older demographic, focusing on improving posture, balance, and core strength, all while being gentle on the joints.

This historical journey of Pilates is not just a story from the past; it's a living, breathing philosophy that continues to evolve and adapt, much like the men who practice it in my gym. As we explore Wall Pilates in this book, we're not just practicing a physical routine; we're embracing a legacy that has transformed millions of lives across generations.

The evolution of Wall Pilates, a fascinating chapter in the larger narrative of physical fitness, is particularly close to my heart as a gym instructor who has journeyed through various realms of exercise and body conditioning. It's a story of innovation, adaptation, and the continuous quest for optimal health and physical well-being.

Wall Pilates, an offshoot of traditional Pilates, emerged as a response to the evolving needs of practitioners, particularly those seeking a more supportive yet challenging workout. In my experience, introducing Wall Pilates into my sessions was a game-changer, especially for men over 40. This demographic often seeks exercises that are gentle on the joints but effective in strengthening and toning the body. Wall Pilates perfectly fits this niche, offering a blend of support and resistance that is not as readily found in traditional Pilates.

The use of the wall in Pilates is a prime example of the adaptability at the core of the discipline. The wall acts as a partner of sorts – providing feedback, resistance, and support. It helps in fine-tuning alignment, enhancing balance, and deepening the engagement of core muscles. For many of my clients, the wall has become an indispensable tool that guides them into better posture and form, which is crucial for those in their 40s and beyond.

As I have integrated Wall Pilates into my routines, I've observed its manifold benefits. It helps build a stronger core, improves balance and coordination, and increases flexibility – all while being low-impact. This is particularly important for older men, as it reduces the risk of injury while still providing a challenging workout. Moreover, it adds an element of variety and challenge to traditional Pilates exercises, keeping the routines fresh and engaging.

Throughout its evolution, Wall Pilates has also been instrumental in breaking down gender stereotypes in the realm of Pilates. Traditionally seen as a female-dominated practice, the addition of the wall and its associated challenges has attracted more men to Pilates, showing them the incredible benefits of this holistic form of exercise.

In my classes, I've seen first-time practitioners transform into dedicated enthusiasts, a testament to the effectiveness and appeal of Wall Pilates. The progression from simple wall-supported stretches to more complex, dynamic movements offers a sense of achievement and progression that is deeply satisfying.

The evolution of Wall Pilates is not just about the physical. It encompasses a journey of mental and emotional growth, echoing the original principles laid down by Joseph Pilates. It's about moving better, feeling better, and living better. As we

Pg. 17

explore this refined version of Pilates, we're not just participating in a fitness trend; we're part of a movement that honors the past while boldly stepping into the future, perfectly tailored for the modern man over 40.

The benefits of Pilates

After years of experience, I've come to appreciate the profound impact of Wall Pilates on men, especially those over 40. The benefits of this specialized form of Pilates are numerous and significant, addressing not just physical fitness but also overall well-being.

Wall Pilates, an adaptation of the traditional Pilates method, integrates the use of a wall as a tool for support, resistance, and feedback. This seemingly simple addition transforms the practice, making it more accessible and beneficial for men, particularly as they age. Men in their 40s and beyond often face unique physical challenges: decreased flexibility, reduced muscle mass, and a higher risk of joint pain and injuries. Wall Pilates directly addresses these issues, offering a safe yet effective way to stay fit and healthy.

One of the most immediate benefits of Wall Pilates that I've observed in my clients is improved posture. As we age, our posture tends to deteriorate due to lifestyle habits and natural changes in the body. The wall acts as a guide in Wall Pilates, helping practitioners understand and maintain proper alignment. This not only improves their appearance but also reduces strain on the spine and joints, leading to fewer aches and pains.

Core strength is another significant benefit. The core is the body's powerhouse – it supports every other part. Wall Pilates exercises are incredibly effective at strengthening the core muscles, which in turn supports better balance, stability, and overall strength. This is crucial for men over 40, as a strong core is essential for preventing falls and maintaining functional fitness.

Furthermore, Wall Pilates enhances flexibility and range of motion. Many men tend to neglect flexibility training, which can lead to stiffness and reduced mobility. The controlled, stretching movements of Wall Pilates, aided by the wall, help in gently extending and flexing muscles, improving flexibility, and decreasing the risk of injury.

In addition to physical benefits, Wall Pilates offers mental and emotional advantages. The focus on controlled, mindful movements promotes a sense of calm and reduces stress. It's a time for men to disconnect from the pressures of daily life, focus on their well-being, and engage in a practice that is both challenging and rejuvenating.

Finally, as men age, the risk of chronic health conditions like heart disease and diabetes increases. Regular exercise, such as Wall Pilates, plays a vital role in managing and preventing these conditions. It's not just about living longer; it's about living better.

Incorporating Wall Pilates into the routines of men over 40 has been a rewarding experience. Witnessing the transformations – stronger bodies, better posture, increased confidence, and a newfound appreciation for holistic fitness – is a testament to the power of this practice. Wall Pilates isn't just an exercise; it's a pathway to a healthier, more balanced life.

Difference between yoga and Pilates

I often encounter questions about the differences between yoga and Pilates. While both practices focus on mind-body connection and involve a series of movements and poses, they are distinct in their origins, techniques, and overall objectives.

Yoga, with its roots in ancient India, is primarily a holistic practice that encompasses physical postures (asanas), breathing techniques (pranayama), and meditation. It aims to achieve a balance between mind, body, and spirit, leading to improved mental, physical, and emotional well-being. Yoga is diverse, with various styles ranging from the physically demanding (like Ashtanga or Vinyasa) to the more gentle and meditative (like Hatha or Yin). As a yoga practitioner, I've observed how it not only enhances flexibility and strength but also instills a sense of peace and mental clarity.

Pilates, on the other hand, was developed in the early 20th century by Joseph Pilates. It is more focused on physical rehabilitation and strengthening. Pilates exercises are designed to improve posture, core strength, muscle tone, and flexibility. The practice emphasizes precise movements and breath control to promote efficient and graceful movement. Pilates can be performed on a mat or with specialized equipment like the Reformer, which provides resistance for muscle strengthening.

In my teaching experience, I've seen that Pilates tends to be more structured than yoga. It focuses on specific exercises performed in a certain order, with a greater emphasis on controlling every aspect of each movement. This control is essential in developing core strength and improving posture. Pilates is particularly beneficial for those looking to rehabilitate injuries, improve athletic performance, or simply maintain a strong and balanced body.

Yoga, with its broader focus on holistic wellness, offers not just physical benefits but also promotes mental and emotional health. It encourages practitioners to explore the depths of their minds and spirits, often incorporating elements of spirituality. The practice of yoga can be a journey of self-discovery, leading to inner peace and mindfulness.

Both yoga and Pilates can be adapted to suit practitioners of all levels and are beneficial in their own ways. As an instructor, I encourage individuals to explore both practices to fully understand their unique benefits. While yoga offers a path to inner peace and physical well-being, Pilates provides a structured approach to physical rehabilitation and strength building. The choice between the two often depends on personal fitness goals, interests, and the need for physical and mental balance.

Why choose wall Pilates

While learning different types of exercises, I've encountered various fitness trends and exercises, but one that stands out distinctively is Wall Pilates. This innovative form of Pilates, which uses a wall as a key prop, offers a unique blend of strength, flexibility, and balance exercises that are particularly beneficial, especially for those seeking a low-impact yet effective workout.

The beauty of Wall Pilates lies in its simplicity and effectiveness. The wall acts as a constant, steady support, making it an excellent tool for beginners and those over 40, who may be more prone to balance issues or injury. It provides stability and feedback, allowing practitioners to perfect their form and deepen their understanding of each movement. This aspect of Wall Pilates has been invaluable in my teaching, as it helps me guide students towards safer and more effective exercises.

Moreover, Wall Pilates is incredibly versatile. It can be adapted to suit various fitness levels and can address specific physical needs or goals. For those looking to build core strength, the wall provides resistance that intensifies traditional Pilates exercises. For others focusing on flexibility or balance, the wall offers support that allows them to stretch further and hold poses longer. This adaptability makes Wall Pilates a suitable choice for a wide range of individuals, including those who are just embarking on their fitness journey or returning from an injury.

Another significant advantage of Wall Pilates, which I often highlight to my clients, is its focus on posture. In today's world, where many of us spend hours hunched over computers or smartphones, a workout that emphasizes proper posture is invaluable. Wall Pilates trains the body to maintain alignment, strengthening the muscles that contribute to a straighter spine and a more upright stance. This not only improves appearance but also reduces the risk of chronic pain and injuries.

Furthermore, Wall Pilates is an excellent tool for mind-body connection. The requirement for concentration and precision in each movement fosters mindfulness, a mental state where one is fully attentive to the present moment. This mindfulness has profound benefits, extending beyond the gym into daily life, enhancing overall well-being.

Incorporating Wall Pilates into my classes has been a transformative experience. I've seen clients develop not just physically, but also gain confidence and a new perspective on what their bodies can achieve, regardless of age or fitness level. Wall Pilates is not just another exercise trend; it's a holistic approach to fitness that respects the body's limitations while challenging it to grow stronger and more flexible. It's a testament to the idea that sometimes, the simplest tools can lead to the most significant changes.

Anatomy of wall Pilates

One of the most enlightening aspects has been understanding and teaching the anatomy for Pilates. This knowledge is not just crucial for performing Pilates effectively but also for appreciating the profound impact it has on the human body.

Anatomy, in the context of Pilates, is about much more than just muscles and bones; it's about understanding how the body moves and functions as a whole. Pilates, with its emphasis on control, precision, and fluid movement, offers a unique window into the intricate workings of our bodies. As an instructor, delving into the anatomy essential for Pilates has not only enhanced my teaching but also deepened my appreciation for this exercise form.

At the core of Pilates is the concept of the 'powerhouse' or the center of the body, which includes the muscles of the abdomen, lower back, hips, and buttocks. These muscles work together to provide support for the spine and pelvis, ensuring stability and balance. Understanding how to engage and strengthen this core area is fundamental to Pilates. In my classes, I emphasize this aspect, educating clients on how strengthening the core can lead to improved posture, better balance, and a reduction in back pain.

Another key anatomical aspect in Pilates is the alignment of the spine. Pilates exercises are designed to promote a neutral spine, which is the natural, healthy position of the spine with its three curves intact. This focus on spinal alignment helps in mitigating issues like chronic back pain and improves overall spinal health. It's fascinating to see clients develop a newfound awareness of their spinal posture, both in and out of the gym.

Flexibility and joint mobility are also integral to Pilates. Understanding the anatomy of the joints and how they move allows for more effective stretching and strengthening exercises. Pilates is particularly beneficial for increasing the range of motion in the hips and shoulders, enhancing overall flexibility and reducing the risk of injuries.

As a gym instructor, my journey into the anatomy for Pilates has been incredibly rewarding. It has allowed me to guide clients more effectively, helping them understand their bodies better and appreciate the benefits of their workouts. Pilates is not just about performing a set of exercises; it's a journey into understanding and appreciating the incredible capabilities and intricacies of the human body. This knowledge empowers individuals to practice Pilates more effectively, leading to better health, improved physical performance, and a greater sense of well-being.

The importance of posture and alignment

Throughout my journey as a gym instructor, I've come to realize the immense importance of posture and alignment in overall fitness and well-being. These are not just buzzwords but fundamental elements that can transform how one feels, moves, and even thinks.

In our daily lives, many of us tend to overlook posture. We slouch at desks, hunch over phones, and neglect our body's alignment. However, the repercussions of poor posture are far-reaching. It can lead to chronic back pain, muscle imbalances, and even affect breathing and digestion. As an instructor, I've seen numerous clients who came in with these issues, unaware that their posture was a significant contributor.

The first step in addressing these problems is awareness. In my sessions, I emphasize understanding and maintaining proper posture. This involves educating clients about the natural curves of the spine and how to align their bodies in both standing and sitting positions. Anatomical alignment of the ears, shoulders, hips, knees, and ankles is a key component of good posture. This might seem simple, but for many, it requires a conscious effort to correct years of bad habits.

Alignment goes hand-in-hand with posture. It's about ensuring that the body parts are correctly positioned relative to each other during movement. In Pilates, and especially in Wall Pilates, alignment is crucial. The exercises are designed to strengthen the muscles that support proper alignment, leading to better balance and movement efficiency. As clients progress in their practice, they often report reduced pain and increased ease in daily activities.

Moreover, good posture and alignment are about more than just physical health. They have a profound impact on confidence and self-perception. There's a noticeable difference in how people carry themselves once they start paying attention to their posture. They stand taller, move better, and exude a sense of confidence. This psychological aspect is a significant part of the fitness journey.

In my teaching, I've found that focusing on posture and alignment has far-reaching benefits. It's not just about looking good; it's about creating a strong foundation for overall health and well-being. This focus is integral to Wall Pilates, where the wall serves as a constant reminder and guide for maintaining proper alignment. As my clients learn to align and carry their bodies correctly, they often find that many of their aches and pains diminish, and they move through life more effortlessly and confidently.

Posture and alignment are, therefore, not just components of a workout routine but essential life skills that enhance one's quality of life.

Mind-body connection in Pilates

I've learned that Pilates is not just about physical strength or flexibility; it's profoundly rooted in the connection between the mind and the body. This mind-body connection is a cornerstone of Pilates, making it a uniquely holistic form of exercise.

Pilates, unlike many other fitness regimes, demands a high level of mental focus and awareness. It's not enough to simply go through the motions; Pilates requires one to be fully present, mentally engaging with each movement. This focus on mindfulness has always intrigued me, and it's something I emphasize in my classes. It's about understanding not just how to move, but also why each movement matters.

One of the first things I teach my clients is the importance of conscious movement. In Pilates, every action is deliberate and controlled, requiring a deep concentration. This conscious control helps in connecting the mind to the body, allowing for a greater understanding and mastery over one's movements. As my clients progress, they often find that they are not just physically stronger, but also more mentally aware of how their bodies move and function.

Breath is another critical aspect of the mind-body connection in Pilates. Joseph Pilates himself emphasized the importance of proper breathing techniques in his method. In my sessions, I guide clients through exercises while focusing on their breathing. This practice of coordinating breath with movement not only enhances the effectiveness of the exercises but also helps in centering the mind, reducing stress, and improving focus.

Furthermore, the mind-body connection in Pilates extends beyond the gym. My clients often report a heightened sense of body awareness in their daily activities. They become more mindful of their posture while sitting, standing, or walking. This constant awareness leads to better movement patterns and, consequently, a reduction in physical discomfort and strain.

In Wall Pilates, this connection is even more pronounced. The wall provides immediate feedback, making it easier for practitioners to be aware of and correct their alignment and posture. It acts as a physical reminder, helping them stay connected to their bodies.

The mind-body connection in Pilates is, for many, a transformative experience. It teaches patience, awareness, and control, not just physically but in all aspects of life. As an instructor, witnessing this transformation is one of the most rewarding aspects of my job. Pilates, in essence, is more than just a form of exercise; it's a pathway to a more mindful, connected, and balanced life.

Breathing techniques in Pilates and their importance

The breathing techniques in Wall Pilates are not just a side note; they are central to the practice's effectiveness and its profound impact on both body and mind.

Breathing, in the context of Wall Pilates, is far more than a mere biological function. It's a tool for enhancing exercise effectiveness, controlling movement, and connecting deeper with oneself. The act of breathing in Wall Pilates is deliberate, synchronized with each movement, creating a rhythm that guides the entire workout. It's this rhythmic, mindful breathing that transforms a physical exercise into a holistic experience.

In my classes, I often start by teaching the basics of Pilates breathing – deep, controlled breaths, inhaled through the nose and exhaled through the mouth. This style of breathing is designed to engage the core muscles, particularly during exhalation, which enhances stability and power in exercises. As my clients learn to coordinate their breath with their movements, they often find a significant increase in the control and efficiency of each exercise. This is especially noticeable in Wall Pilates, where precision and control are paramount.

Moreover, the breathing techniques in Wall Pilates are not just about physical benefits. They play a crucial role in mental focus and relaxation. The concentrated effort to breathe deeply and rhythmically requires a level of mindfulness that brings clients into the present moment, clearing the mind of distractions. This focus is incredibly beneficial for stress reduction. Many of my clients have shared how this focused breathing has helped them manage stress and anxiety, both during workouts and in their everyday lives.

The wall in Wall Pilates adds a unique dimension to these breathing techniques. It acts as a physical reminder, a support that clients can feel and align their movements and breaths against. This connection to the wall helps in maintaining a steady breathing rhythm, making the exercises more effective and the mind more centered.

In essence, breathing in Wall Pilates is a bridge between the physical and the mental. It enhances the effectiveness of the exercises while also fostering a sense of inner calm and mindfulness. As an instructor, guiding clients through this process is deeply fulfilling. Witnessing how they harness their breath to gain strength, control, and peace is a testament to the power of Wall Pilates. It's more than just a workout; it's a practice that nurtures both the body and the soul.

Building from basics

One of the most rewarding aspects has been guiding clients through the progression from basic to more advanced levels, especially in the realm of Wall Pilates. This transition, often referred to as "Building on the Basics," is a crucial phase where foundational skills are expanded into more challenging and complex movements.

Starting with the basics in Wall Pilates, clients learn fundamental postures and movements, focusing on correct form, breathing, and alignment. These foundational exercises are the building blocks of the practice. They establish muscle memory, core strength, and an understanding of how the body moves and balances. In my sessions, I emphasize mastering these basics, as they set the groundwork for all future progressions.

However, the journey doesn't stop there. Building on the basics is where the real transformation begins. Once my clients are comfortable with the foundational exercises, we gradually introduce more challenging variations. These advanced movements require greater strength, flexibility, and control, pushing the body and mind to new limits.

This progression is not just about increasing physical intensity; it's about deepening the connection with one's body. As clients move to more advanced exercises, they develop a heightened awareness of their physical capabilities and limitations. They learn to listen to their bodies, understanding when to push harder and when to pull back. This self-awareness is a critical component of physical fitness, especially for men over 40, who need to be mindful of their body's signals.

In Wall Pilates, the wall serves as a constant companion in this journey of progression. As exercises become more complex, the wall provides feedback and support, allowing clients to explore their limits safely. It's an invaluable tool for enhancing balance, refining posture, and intensifying core engagement.

Building on the basics is also a journey of mental and emotional growth. With each new challenge, clients build not just physical strength but also mental resilience. They learn the value of persistence, patience, and dedication. The satisfaction of mastering a difficult move after weeks or months of practice is immensely rewarding, both for the client and for me as an instructor.

In summary, "Building on the Basics" in Wall Pilates is about more than just moving to advanced exercises. It's a holistic journey that involves physical, mental, and emotional development. It's about pushing boundaries, exploring potential, and embracing the continuous journey of self-improvement. As clients progress, they not only enhance their physical fitness but also gain a deeper appreciation for what their bodies and minds can achieve.

Maintaining consistency and motivation

In my experience as a gym instructor, I've learned that one of the biggest challenges people face in their fitness journey is maintaining consistency and motivation. This is especially true in practices like Wall Pilates, where progress can be gradual and demands regular commitment.

The key to maintaining consistency, as I often tell my clients, lies in setting realistic goals and establishing a routine. It's about making exercise a regular part of your life, rather than something you do sporadically. In Wall Pilates, this might mean setting aside specific days and times for practice, ensuring it becomes as habitual as brushing your teeth. The wall serves as a physical anchor, a reminder of the commitment to one's health and well-being.

But establishing a routine is only part of the equation. Keeping motivation high is equally important and often more challenging. One strategy I've found effective is helping clients track their progress. In Wall Pilates, this could involve noting improvements in flexibility, balance, or core strength over time. When clients see how far they've come, it fuels their motivation to continue.

Another motivation booster is varying the routine. While consistency in practice is important, monotony can be a motivation killer. Introducing new exercises, changing the sequence, or setting new challenges within the Wall Pilates regimen keeps the sessions fresh and engaging. It's exciting for clients to tackle new movements or perfect ones they found challenging previously.

Community support also plays a crucial role in maintaining motivation. In my classes, I foster a supportive and encouraging environment. When clients see others working towards similar goals, it creates a sense of camaraderie and collective motivation. Sharing struggles and successes within the group makes the journey less solitary and more enjoyable.

Furthermore, I emphasize the importance of recognizing and celebrating small victories. In the realm of fitness, progress can be incremental, and it's easy to overlook small improvements.

Acknowledging these achievements, whether it's holding a pose a few seconds longer or executing a movement with better form, can be incredibly motivating.

Lastly, I encourage clients to connect their fitness goals to broader life goals. For instance, improving balance and core strength in Wall Pilates might be linked to playing sports better or enjoying active playtime with grandchildren. This connection often provides a deeper, more personal motivation that goes beyond physical appearance or ability.

In conclusion, maintaining consistency and motivation in Wall Pilates, or any fitness endeavor, requires a multifaceted approach. It's about setting routines, tracking progress, introducing variety, fostering community, celebrating small victories, and connecting fitness to personal life goals. As an instructor, guiding clients through this process and seeing them stay committed and motivated is one of the most rewarding aspects of my work.

Wall Pilates for rehabilitation

Throughout my career as a gym instructor, I've come to recognize the exceptional value of Wall Pilates in the realm of rehabilitation. This method, with its unique blend of support and resistance offered by the wall, provides an ideal environment for those recovering from injuries or dealing with chronic pain, especially in the over-40 age group.

Rehabilitation is a delicate process, one that requires a careful balance between challenging the body and respecting its current limitations. Wall Pilates fits perfectly into this delicate balance. The wall serves as a sturdy support, offering stability and safety, which is crucial for anyone in the process of rehabilitating. It allows individuals to perform exercises with a lower risk of injury, giving them the confidence to engage in movements they might otherwise avoid.

In my practice, I've seen how Wall Pilates can be particularly beneficial for those recovering from back injuries or dealing with chronic back pain, common issues among older adults. The exercises, focusing on core strength and spinal alignment, help in strengthening the muscles that support the back, thereby reducing pain and improving overall back health. The controlled, gentle movements of Wall Pilates allow for strengthening without straining, making it an ideal choice for rehabilitation.

Moreover, the versatility of Wall Pilates means exercises can be easily modified to suit various rehabilitation needs. Whether it's adjusting the intensity, range of motion, or duration, the exercises can be tailored to individual requirements. This flexibility ensures a personalized approach to rehabilitation, which is key to effective recovery.

Another aspect of Wall Pilates that makes it suitable for rehabilitation is its focus on whole-body awareness and control. Rehabilitation isn't just about healing a specific injury; it's about retraining the body to move in a way that prevents future injuries. Wall Pilates encourages this retraining, teaching individuals to move with greater mindfulness and efficiency.

Furthermore, rehabilitation can be as much a mental challenge as it is physical. Wall Pilates, with its emphasis on mind-body connection, helps individuals in rehab to stay mentally engaged and positive. The focus required for the exercises, combined with the calming effects of controlled breathing, can be incredibly beneficial for mental well-being during the recovery process.

Incorporating Wall Pilates into rehabilitation programs has been a rewarding aspect of my work as a gym instructor. It's gratifying to witness the gradual, yet profound, progress of individuals as they use Wall Pilates to overcome physical challenges and regain strength, flexibility, and confidence. This method is not just about recovery; it's about empowering individuals to take control of their healing journey and emerge stronger and more resilient.

Wall Pilates for back health

In my years as a gym instructor, focusing on Pilates for back health has been a cornerstone of my approach to fitness, especially considering the prevalence of back issues in today's society. Pilates, with its emphasis on core strength, flexibility, and postural alignment, offers remarkable benefits for maintaining and enhancing back health, which I have witnessed firsthand in many of my clients.

Back health is a complex and multifaceted issue. Poor posture, sedentary lifestyles, and incorrect movement patterns often contribute to back pain and discomfort, which can significantly impact quality of life. Pilates addresses these root causes by focusing on building a strong core – the abdominal, lower back, and pelvic muscles. A strong core is essential for supporting the spine, maintaining good posture, and preventing injuries.

In Pilates, we don't just work on isolated muscle groups; the exercises are designed to engage the entire body in a balanced way. This holistic approach ensures that no single part is overworked or neglected, promoting overall muscular balance and spinal alignment. As an instructor, I guide my clients through exercises that strengthen the back and teach them how to engage their core muscles effectively. This not only alleviates existing back pain but also helps in preventing future issues.

Another key aspect of Pilates for back health is improving flexibility and range of motion. Tight muscles, particularly in the hips and hamstrings, can pull on the spine and lead to discomfort. Pilates exercises gently stretch and strengthen these areas, reducing tension and promoting a more aligned and pain-free back.

Moreover, Pilates encourages awareness of body mechanics and posture. Through regular practice, my clients become more mindful of how they sit, stand, and move throughout the day. This increased awareness is crucial for avoiding the habits that often lead to back problems.

I have seen remarkable transformations in clients who have turned to Pilates for back health. They often report reduced pain, increased mobility, and a greater ability to engage in daily activities without discomfort. For many, Pilates becomes more than a workout routine; it's a pathway to a more pain-free, active lifestyle.

In summary, Pilates offers a comprehensive approach to back health, addressing the underlying causes of back pain through a combination of strength, flexibility, and postural training. As a gym instructor, it's been incredibly rewarding to help clients strengthen their backs, improve their posture, and enhance their overall well-being through Pilates.

Common male injuries

In my career as a gym instructor, one aspect I've frequently encountered is the prevalence of certain injuries among men, particularly as they age. Addressing these common male injuries is not just about rehabilitation; it's about understanding their causes and working towards prevention.

From my observations and interactions, I've noticed that men often suffer from injuries related to overuse, improper technique, or lack of flexibility. These include issues like lower back pain, shoulder injuries, knee problems, and muscle strains. The reasons vary, ranging from sports-related activities to the stresses of daily life or even the natural aging process.

In tackling these injuries, my approach has always been twofold: rehabilitation and prevention. For those already dealing with injuries, the key is to provide exercises that help in recovery without exacerbating the issue. This is where tailored workouts like Wall Pilates come into play. The support of the wall allows for controlled, low-impact movements that focus on strengthening and flexibility, crucial for recovery. For instance, exercises targeting the core and lower back can alleviate back pain, while shoulder and arm exercises can aid in recovering from shoulder injuries.

Prevention, however, is equally important. Educating men on proper exercise techniques and body mechanics is vital. Many injuries result from incorrect form or pushing the body beyond its limits. In my classes, I emphasize the importance of listening to one's body, understanding the difference between pushing oneself healthily and going too far. This education is a cornerstone of injury prevention.

Flexibility and strength training are also key components. Often, men focus heavily on strength and neglect flexibility, leading to muscle imbalances and increased injury risk. Incorporating stretching and exercises that enhance range of motion is essential. Pilates, with its focus on controlled, fluid movements, is excellent for building both strength and flexibility.

Lastly, consistency in practice plays a crucial role. Regular exercise helps maintain muscle strength, flexibility, and joint health, which are all crucial for injury prevention. As an instructor, I encourage a consistent routine that includes a mix of cardiovascular, strength, and flexibility training.

In summary, addressing common male injuries in the gym is about more than just dealing with the injury at hand. It's about adopting a comprehensive approach that includes rehabilitation, education on proper techniques, a balance of strength and flexibility training, and maintaining a consistent exercise routine. Through this approach, I aim to help men not only recover from their injuries but also build resilience against future issues.

Wall Pilates and weight loss

In my experience as a gym instructor, a common goal among many clients is weight loss. While there are various methods to achieve this, one that has consistently shown positive results is Wall Pilates. This might come as a surprise to some, as Pilates, particularly Wall Pilates, is often not the first thing that comes to mind when thinking about weight loss. However, its effectiveness lies in its approach to overall fitness and body conditioning.

Wall Pilates, a variant of traditional Pilates that utilizes a wall for support and resistance, offers a unique combination of muscle strengthening, toning, and flexibility exercises. While it might seem less intense than high-impact cardiovascular workouts, Wall Pilates can be quite effective in aiding weight loss and body shaping, especially when combined with other healthy lifestyle choices.

One of the key aspects of Wall Pilates that aids in weight loss is its focus on building lean muscle mass. Muscle tissue burns more calories than fat, even at rest. Therefore, by increasing muscle mass through Wall Pilates exercises, the body becomes more efficient at burning calories. This is particularly beneficial for men over 40, as muscle mass naturally begins to decrease with age. Maintaining muscle through targeted exercises helps keep the metabolism active, aiding in weight management.

Moreover, Wall Pilates improves core strength and posture, which can have a surprising effect on weight loss. A strong core and good posture enhance the efficiency of movements and workouts. Clients often find that as their core strength improves, they perform better in other exercises and activities, leading to increased calorie burn.

Another factor is the holistic approach of Wall Pilates. It encourages mindfulness and body awareness. This mindfulness can translate into better eating habits and lifestyle choices, which are crucial components of weight loss. Many of my clients have reported that their Pilates practice has helped them develop a more conscious relationship with their bodies, leading to healthier eating and lifestyle habits.

Additionally, the versatility of Wall Pilates means it can be adapted to various fitness levels and can be made more challenging as one progresses. This adaptability keeps the workouts interesting and challenging, ensuring that clients continue to see results over time.

In conclusion, while Wall Pilates may not be the quickest method for weight loss, its comprehensive approach to building muscle, improving posture, and enhancing overall fitness makes it a valuable tool in a weight loss journey. When combined with a balanced diet and other physical activities, Wall Pilates can significantly contribute to achieving and maintaining a healthy weight, especially for men over 40.

Proper dieting for a better result

In my role as a gym instructor, one question I frequently encounter from those practicing Wall Pilates – or any form of exercise, for that matter – is about the right diet to complement their workout routine. Nutrition plays a crucial role in maximizing the benefits of Wall Pilates, particularly for those looking to improve muscle tone, increase strength, and enhance overall well-being.

Wall Pilates, with its emphasis on core strength, flexibility, and balance, demands a diet that supports muscle recovery, energy, and general health. The key is to find a balance of nutrients that fuels the body both for the workouts and for recovery afterward. This means a diet rich in lean proteins, complex carbohydrates, healthy fats, and, of course, plenty of vitamins and minerals from fruits and vegetables.

Lean protein is essential for muscle repair and growth. For my clients engaged in Wall Pilates, I often suggest incorporating a variety of protein sources like chicken, fish, beans, and legumes into their diet. These foods help in muscle recovery, especially after a strenuous workout.

Complex carbohydrates are also vital. They provide the energy needed to perform Pilates exercises effectively. Whole grains, such as brown rice, quinoa, and whole wheat products, offer sustained energy, keeping you fueled throughout your workout and the day.

Healthy fats, found in foods like avocados, nuts, and olive oil, are also important. They support overall health, reduce inflammation, and aid in the absorption of certain vitamins.

Hydration is another critical element. Staying well-hydrated is essential for overall health and helps ensure that the body functions optimally during exercise. I always remind my clients to drink plenty of water before, during, and after their Pilates sessions.

Lastly, fruits and vegetables are non-negotiable. They're packed with vitamins, minerals, and antioxidants that support overall health, reduce muscle soreness, and aid in recovery. A diet rich in a variety of colorful fruits and vegetables ensures that you're getting a wide range of nutrients essential for good health.

A balanced diet that incorporates these elements supports the physical demands of Wall Pilates and contributes to overall health and wellness. It's not just about eating for a workout; it's about nurturing your body with the right nutrients for optimal health and performance. As a gym instructor, guiding my clients in their nutritional choices is as important as guiding them in their workouts. The right diet can significantly enhance the benefits of Wall Pilates, leading to better results and a healthier lifestyle.

CHAPTER 2: HOW TO GET STARTED WITH WALL PILATES

Starting with Wall Pilates, particularly for those new to the practice or returning to exercise after a break, can be both exciting and a bit daunting. In my journey as a gym instructor, guiding beginners through this process has been a rewarding experience. Wall Pilates, with its unique use of the wall for support and resistance, offers a gentle yet effective way to build strength, flexibility, and balance.

The first step in getting started with Wall Pilates is understanding the basics of Pilates itself. I often begin by explaining the core principles of Pilates - control, concentration, precision, breath, and flow. These principles are the foundation of all Pilates exercises, including those performed using the wall. It's important for beginners to grasp these concepts as they form the basis for a successful practice.

Next, I introduce my clients to the wall. The wall is a versatile tool in Wall Pilates. It can be used for support, helping beginners to perform exercises with proper form and alignment. It also adds resistance to exercises, making them more challenging. I show my clients how to use the wall effectively - how to stand or lean against it, how to use it for balance, and how to incorporate it into different exercises.

We then move on to basic exercises. I start with simple movements that focus on core engagement, posture, and balance. These might include wall-assisted squats, wall push-ups, or leg slides. These exercises are designed to build confidence and familiarity with the practice. The emphasis is always on quality of movement rather than quantity.

Breathing techniques are another crucial aspect of Wall Pilates that I introduce early on. Proper breathing helps in executing movements with greater control and efficiency. It also enhances concentration and focus.

Safety is a key consideration, especially for beginners. I ensure my clients are aware of their body's limits and encourage them to listen to their bodies, avoiding pushing too hard too soon. I also remind them of the importance of a proper warm-up and cool-down in each session.

Finally, consistency is key in Wall Pilates. I encourage beginners to practice regularly. Consistency helps in building and maintaining the strength, flexibility, and balance gained through Pilates.

In summary, getting started with Wall Pilates involves understanding the basics of Pilates, learning how to use the wall effectively, starting with simple exercises, focusing on proper breathing techniques, and practicing consistently. As an instructor, guiding beginners through this journey is about ensuring a safe, enjoyable, and effective world of Wall Pilates.

Important equipments and Pilate space

In my journey as a gym instructor, I've found that setting up the right environment and having the essential equipment are crucial for an effective Wall

Pilates session. While Wall Pilates doesn't require a lot of equipment or a vast space, the quality and appropriateness of what you use can significantly enhance the experience and effectiveness of the workout.

Firstly, the space for Wall Pilates needs to be adequate. It doesn't have to be large, but it should be enough to allow free movement. A clear wall space is essential – it's the core of Wall Pilates. This wall should be free of obstructions, providing a solid, flat surface to lean against, push off from, or balance with. The right environment should be calming and free from distractions, allowing for focus and concentration during the session. In my gym, I have a dedicated area for Wall Pilates with minimalistic decor and a tranquil atmosphere, which helps clients to focus inward and connect with their bodies.

When it comes to equipment, one of the beauties of Wall Pilates is its simplicity. The primary 'equipment' is the wall itself. However, a few additional items can enhance the practice. A good-quality yoga mat is one of these essentials. It provides cushioning and grip, which are important for both comfort and safety, especially when performing floor exercises.

Another useful piece of equipment is resistance bands. These bands can be used for a variety of exercises, adding resistance to strengthen and tone muscles. They are particularly useful for adding intensity to arm and leg exercises in Wall Pilates.

For those looking to deepen their practice, a stability ball can be a valuable addition. It can be used against the wall for exercises like wall squats or pelvic tilts, adding an extra challenge to balance and core stability.

In terms of attire, comfortable and non-restrictive clothing is essential. Clients should wear something that allows them to move freely and doesn't get in the way. Footwear is usually not necessary; most people prefer to do Pilates barefoot or in socks for better grip.

In summary, the essentials for Wall Pilates are quite straightforward – a clear wall space, a good mat, and optionally, some resistance bands and a stability ball. The simplicity of equipment and space required for Wall Pilates makes it an accessible form of exercise, yet the possibilities for strengthening, toning, and improving flexibility are immense. As an instructor, part of my role is to help clients make the most of these tools, guiding them through exercises that transform their physical and mental well-being.

Important safety precautions

In my experience as a gym instructor, I've always placed a strong emphasis on safety, especially when it comes to exercises like Wall Pilates. While Pilates is generally a low-impact and safe form of exercise, certain precautions are necessary to ensure a risk-free and beneficial workout, particularly for individuals who might be new to the practice or have specific health concerns.

One of the fundamental safety tips I impart to my clients is the importance of understanding their own bodies. It's crucial to be aware of personal limits and not push beyond what feels comfortable. This is especially true for men over 40, who might be dealing with joint sensitivities or other age-related physical changes. I encourage them to listen to their bodies and stop immediately if they feel any pain or discomfort.

Proper form and technique are vital in Wall Pilates. Incorrect form can lead to strain or injury, particularly in the back and neck. As an instructor, I closely monitor my clients' postures and movements, correcting them when necessary. For beginners, I often start with basic exercises, gradually increasing the difficulty as they become more comfortable and their form improves.

The wall, being an integral part of Wall Pilates, must be used correctly. It's important to ensure that the wall used is stable and free of any objects that could cause injury. When leaning or pushing against the wall, the force should be controlled and evenly distributed to avoid undue stress on any part of the body.

Another key aspect of safety is the use of equipment. If using resistance bands or stability balls, I make sure my clients know how to use them correctly. Equipment should be in good condition and appropriate for the exercise. For instance,

Pg. 62

resistance bands should be free from tears or frays to prevent snapping.

Warm-ups and cool-downs are a non-negotiable part of the routine. I always start with a warm-up to prepare the body for exercise, gradually increasing the heart rate and loosening the muscles and joints. Similarly, cooling down with stretches after a session helps in preventing muscle stiffness and soreness.

Lastly, I advise clients to stay hydrated and avoid overexertion. Regular sips of water throughout the session help in maintaining hydration, and breaks are encouraged whenever needed.

In summary, safety in Wall Pilates revolves around understanding and respecting one's body, maintaining proper form, correctly using the wall and any equipment, and ensuring a thorough warm-up and cool-down. These practices are essential for a safe and effective workout, helping to prevent injury and maximize the benefits of Pilates. As an instructor, guiding my clients through this process safely is of utmost importance and one of the most rewarding aspects of my work.

Fitness levels

In my journey as a gym instructor, a crucial step before starting any fitness program, including Wall Pilates, is assessing an individual's fitness level. This assessment is not about judging or comparing but understanding where a person is starting from to tailor a workout plan that is both safe and effective.

The process begins with a conversation. I talk with my clients about their exercise history, lifestyle, and any health concerns. This discussion provides insight into their physical activity levels and any potential limitations. For men over 40, it's especially important to consider factors like joint health, flexibility, and any chronic conditions such as heart disease or arthritis.

Next, I observe their basic movements. Simple actions like walking, bending, and sitting can tell a lot about a person's balance, flexibility, and posture. In Wall Pilates, these elements are crucial as they impact how well an individual will be able to perform the exercises. Observing these movements helps in identifying any imbalances or areas that need special attention.

I also conduct a few basic fitness tests. These might include a core strength test, a flexibility test, and a balance test. For example, holding a plank position can give a good indication of core strength, while a simple toe-touch test can assess hamstring and lower back flexibility. Balance can be evaluated through exercises like standing on one leg. These tests are not meant to be challenging but rather to provide a baseline of the individual's current fitness.

Another important aspect is discussing goals. Understanding what my clients hope to achieve helps in creating a program that aligns with their aspirations, whether it's improving strength, flexibility, balance, or overall fitness. This goal-setting is a collaborative process, ensuring the goals are realistic and achievable.

Once the assessment is complete, I use this information to design a personalized Wall Pilates program. This program takes into account their current fitness level, any physical limitations, and their goals. The idea is to start at a comfortable level and gradually increase the intensity and complexity of the exercises.

In summary, assessing fitness levels is a vital part of starting any fitness regimen. It's about creating a strong foundation on which to build a successful and sustainable fitness journey. As an instructor, guiding my clients through this assessment process is key to helping them achieve their fitness goals safely and effectively.

Who should use and who should avoid the wall Pilates

When considering who should embrace or avoid Wall Pilates, especially for men, it's important to understand that while Wall Pilates is a versatile and generally low-impact form of exercise, it may not be suitable for everyone. As a gym instructor, I've seen a wide range of clients benefit from Wall Pilates, but

I've also advised certain individuals to avoid it or to seek medical advice before starting.

Who Should Use Wall Pilates:

1. Men Over 40 Seeking Low-Impact Exercise: Wall Pilates is excellent for older men who need a workout that's gentle on the joints but effective in building strength, flexibility, and balance.

2. Those Looking to Improve Posture and Core Strength: Men who spend long hours at a desk or have sedentary lifestyles can benefit immensely from Wall Pilates. It's effective in strengthening the core and improving posture.

3. Individuals Recovering from Certain Injuries: Under professional guidance, men recovering from specific injuries, particularly related to the back, shoulders, or knees, may find Wall Pilates beneficial due to its controlled, strengthening movements.

4. Men Seeking to Enhance Flexibility: Those looking to improve their flexibility, including athletes and fitness enthusiasts, can benefit from the stretching and lengthening aspects of Wall Pilates.

5. Anyone Looking for Mind-Body Exercise: Men interested in exercises that combine physical fitness with mental well-being may find Wall Pilates particularly rewarding.

Who Should Avoid Wall Pilates:

1. Individuals with Severe Osteoporosis: Those with severe osteoporosis or at high risk of fractures should avoid Wall Pilates due to the risks associated with certain movements.

2. Men with Advanced Cardiovascular Diseases: Those with advanced heart conditions should seek medical advice before starting Wall Pilates, as it might not be the most suitable form of exercise for them.

3. Those Recovering from Certain Surgeries: Men who have recently undergone major surgeries, especially in the back, abdomen, or joints, should avoid Wall Pilates until fully recovered and cleared by a medical professional.

4. Individuals with Acute Hernia: Those with an acute hernia may find some movements in Wall Pilates aggravate their condition.

5. People Experiencing Severe Pain or Discomfort: Anyone experiencing severe pain or discomfort during exercise should avoid Wall Pilates until the cause of the pain is identified and addressed.

In summary, while Wall Pilates is adaptable and beneficial for many, it's not universally suitable. Men considering this form of exercise should evaluate their physical condition, consult with healthcare providers if necessary, and ideally start under the guidance of a qualified instructor.

CHAPTER 3: WARMUP EXERCISES

Jogging in Place

Jogging in Place is a simple, yet effective cardiovascular exercise that can be performed virtually anywhere without the need for any special equipment. This exercise is excellent for warming up the body before more intense workouts, improving cardiovascular health, and boosting endurance. It's a versatile activity suitable for all fitness levels, offering the benefits of jogging without the need for a large space or running track.

Instructions for Jogging in Place

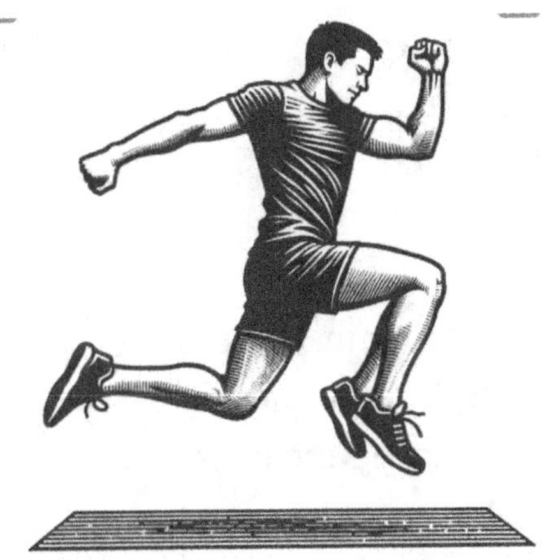

1. Starting Position: Stand with your feet hip-width apart. Keep your back straight, shoulders relaxed, and look straight ahead.

2. Movement: Begin by lifting your heels off the ground, and start jogging lightly on the spot. Your arms should naturally swing in coordination with the opposite leg's movement.

3. Arm Movement: Bend your elbows at about a 90-degree angle. As your left knee comes up, your right arm should swing forward and vice versa. This arm movement is key to maintaining balance and rhythm.

4. Foot Landing: Land softly on the balls of your feet to reduce impact on your joints. The movement should feel natural and light, keeping the pace steady.

5. Breathing: Maintain a steady breathing pattern. Inhale and exhale rhythmically to ensure a constant flow of oxygen during the exercise.

Number of Sets and Repetitions

- ☐ - Beginners: Start with 1 to 2 sets of 30 seconds to 1 minute each. Gradually increase as your endurance improves.
- ☐ - Intermediate: Aim for 2 to 3 sets of 2 to 3 minutes each.
- ☐ - Advanced: Challenge yourself with longer durations, such as 3 to 5 sets of 3 to 5 minutes each.

Remember, the key to jogging in place is consistency and gradually increasing the intensity. It's a great exercise to get your heart rate up, improve your cardiovascular health, and build stamina over time.

Jumping Jacks

Jumping Jacks are a classic, dynamic exercise that combines cardiovascular conditioning with full-body toning. This exercise is excellent for warming up your muscles, increasing your heart rate, and improving coordination and stamina. One of the greatest advantages of Jumping Jacks is their simplicity and the fact that they can be performed almost anywhere without any special equipment.

Instructions for Jumping Jacks

1. Starting Position: Stand upright with your legs together and arms at your sides. Keep your back straight and your gaze forward.

2. Movement: Jump up, spreading your legs wider than shoulder-width apart while simultaneously raising your arms above your head. Your body should form an 'X' shape at the peak of the jump.

3. Return Movement: Quickly jump back to the starting position, bringing your legs together and your arms back to your sides.

4. Breathing: Inhale as you jump and spread your limbs, and exhale as you return to the starting position. Keep your breathing steady and rhythmic to maintain endurance.

5. Pace: Maintain a fast yet controlled pace. The motion should be continuous, with one jump flowing into the next.

Number of Sets and Repetitions

- ☐ - Beginners: Start with 1 to 2 sets of 10 to 15 repetitions each. Focus on form and coordination.
- ☐ - Intermediate: Increase to 2 to 3 sets of 20 to 30 repetitions.
- ☐ - Advanced: Aim for longer sets, such as 3 to 5 sets of 50 or more repetitions, or incorporate them into high-intensity interval training (HIIT).

Jumping Jacks are a great way to boost your cardiovascular health and improve muscle tone. They can be easily integrated into any workout routine, offering a quick and effective way to get your heart pumping.

Arm Circles

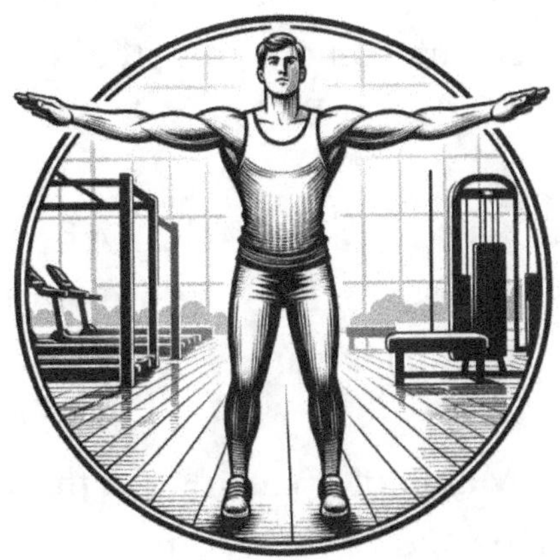

Arm Circles are a fundamental exercise that targets the shoulders, triceps, and upper back. They are an excellent way to warm up these areas, improve shoulder mobility, and build muscle endurance. Arm Circles are versatile and can be easily adjusted to suit any fitness level, making them a great addition to both low-impact warm-up routines and more intense workout sessions.

Instructions for Arm Circles

1. Starting Position: Place your feet shoulder-width apart as you stand. Raise your arms to shoulder height and extend them straight out to the sides.

2. Movement - Forward Circles: Begin circling your arms forward in small, controlled motions. Ensure that the movement comes from the shoulder joint, keeping the rest of your body stable.

3. Movement - Backward Circles: After completing the forward circles, reverse the direction and start circling your arms backward.

4. Breathing: Maintain a steady, rhythmic breathing pattern. Inhale and exhale smoothly to keep a consistent pace and ensure a steady flow of oxygen.

5. Posture: Keep your back straight, core engaged, and shoulders down and relaxed to avoid unnecessary tension in the neck.

Number of Sets and Repetitions

- ☐ - Beginners: Start with 1 to 2 sets of 10 to 15 circles in each direction. Focus on form and smooth motion.
- ☐ - Intermediate: Increase to 2 to 3 sets of 20 to 30 circles in each direction.
- ☐ - Advanced: For a more intense workout, aim for longer sets or incorporate hand weights to increase resistance. Try 3 to 5 sets of 40 or more circles in each direction.

Arm Circles are a simple yet effective exercise for improving upper body strength and flexibility. They can be performed almost anywhere and easily integrated into any fitness routine, providing a quick and efficient way to warm up and tone the muscles in your shoulders and arms.

<u>Lunges</u>

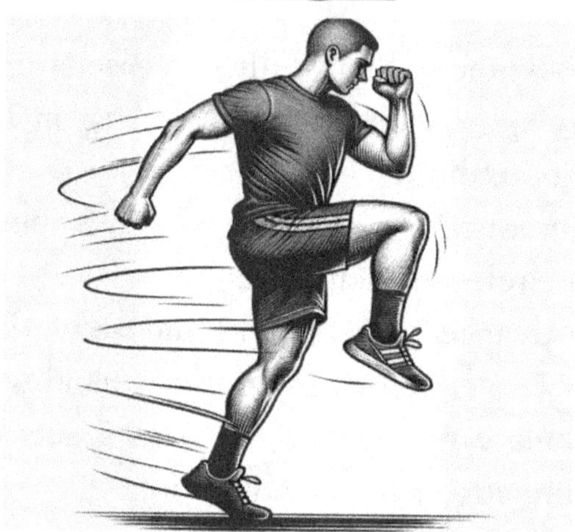

Lunges are a fundamental strength exercise that targets the lower body, focusing on the quadriceps, glutes, and hamstrings. They are incredibly effective for building lower body strength, improving balance and coordination, and enhancing core stability. Lunges are versatile, can be done with or without weights, and are suitable for all fitness levels.

Instructions for Lunges

1. Starting Position: Stand tall with your feet hip-width apart. Keep your arms at your sides or place your hands on your hips for balance.

2. Movement: Step forward with one foot, about two feet ahead of the other. Lower your body towards the ground by bending both knees. Aim for a 90-degree angle in both the front and back knee, ensuring your front knee is aligned with your ankle, not pushing over your toes.

3. Lowering Phase: Lower your body until your back knee is just above the ground. Keep your upper body straight and core engaged.

4. Upward Movement: Push through the heel of your front foot to return to the starting position.

5. Alternate Legs: Repeat the movement with the opposite leg. This counts as one repetition.

6. Breathing: Inhale as you lower your body and exhale as you push back up to the starting position.

Number of Sets and Repetitions

- ☐ - Beginners: Start with 1 to 2 sets of 8 to 10 lunges on each leg. Focus on form and balance.
- ☐ - Intermediate: Perform 2 to 3 sets of 12 to 15 lunges per leg.
- ☐ - Advanced: Increase the challenge by adding weights, doing walking lunges, or increasing the number of sets and repetitions.

Lunges are an excellent exercise for those looking to strengthen and tone their lower body. They not only improve muscle endurance but also contribute to better functional movement in daily life. Remember to keep your movements controlled and maintain proper form to maximize the benefits and prevent injury.

Shoulder Shrugs

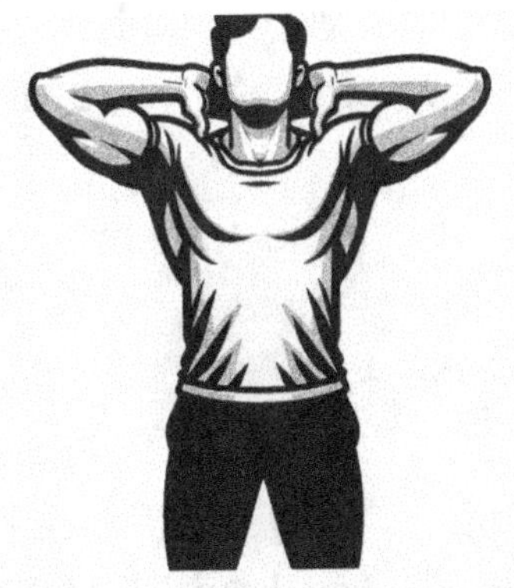

Shoulder Shrugs are a simple yet effective exercise aimed at strengthening and toning the upper trapezius muscles, which are located in the upper back and extend over to the neck. This exercise is excellent for improving shoulder mobility and posture, and it's particularly beneficial for those who spend long hours at a desk or in front of a computer. Shoulder Shrugs can help alleviate tension and stiffness in the neck and shoulder area.

Instructions for Shoulder Shrugs

1. Starting Position: Maintain a hip-width distance between your feet. At your sides, let your arms rest loosely.

2. Movement: Slowly lift your shoulders up towards your ears as high as you can. Keep the movement controlled, focusing on the upward shrug.

3. Hold and Lower: Hold the shrug at the top for a moment, then slowly lower your shoulders back to the starting position.

4. Breathing: Inhale as you lift your shoulders up, and exhale as you lower them back down.

5. Posture: Keep your neck relaxed and your back straight throughout the exercise. Avoid rolling your shoulders forward or backward as you shrug.

Number of Sets and Repetitions

- ☐ - Beginners: Start with 2 sets of 10 to 12 repetitions. Focus on form and the full range of motion.
- ☐ - Intermediate: Perform 3 sets of 12 to 15 repetitions.
- ☐ - Advanced: Increase the challenge by holding weights in your hands during the exercise. Aim for 3 to 5 sets of 15 to 20 repetitions.

Shoulder Shrugs are an excellent way to strengthen and tone your upper back and neck muscles, which are crucial for good posture and shoulder health. They are easy to perform and can be done anywhere, making them a convenient exercise for both gym and home workouts. Remember to keep the motion controlled and focus on engaging the muscles during the shrug.

Torso Twists

Torso Twists are a beneficial exercise focused on improving the flexibility and mobility of the spine and core muscles. This exercise is excellent for loosening up the muscles around the spine, enhancing rotational mobility, and strengthening the core. It's a popular movement in many workout routines because of its simplicity and effectiveness, especially for those seeking to improve their overall spinal health and posture.

Instructions for Torso Twists

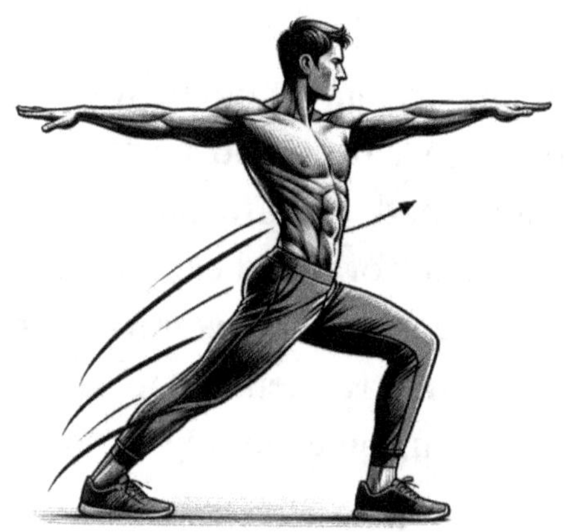

1. Starting Position: Place your feet shoulder-width apart as you stand. Raise your arms shoulder-high and out to the sides.

2. Movement: Keeping your hips facing forward, twist your torso to the right as far as comfortably possible. Your head should follow the direction of the twist, and your arms should remain extended.

3. Hold and Return: Hold the twist for a moment, feeling the stretch along your spine and sides. Then, gently return to the starting position.

4. Repeat on the Other Side: Repeat the twist to the left side. This completes one repetition.

5. Breathing: Inhale in the starting position. Exhale as you twist, and inhale as you return to the center.

6. Posture: Keep your posture upright and avoid bending forward or backward. Controlled and seamless movement is required.

Number of Sets and Repetitions

- ☐ - Beginners: Start with 2 sets of 8 to 10 repetitions on each side. Focus on the smoothness of the movement.
- ☐ - Intermediate: Perform 3 sets of 12 to 15 repetitions on each side.
- ☐ - Advanced: Increase the intensity by holding a light weight in your hands or increasing the number of sets and repetitions.

Torso Twists are a simple yet effective way to improve your core strength and spinal flexibility. This exercise is particularly beneficial for those who spend long hours sitting, as it helps counteract the stiffness associated with a sedentary lifestyle. Remember to perform each twist with control and to respect your body's limits.

CHAPTER 4: CORE STRENGTHENING EXERCISES

Wall Sit Leg Lifts

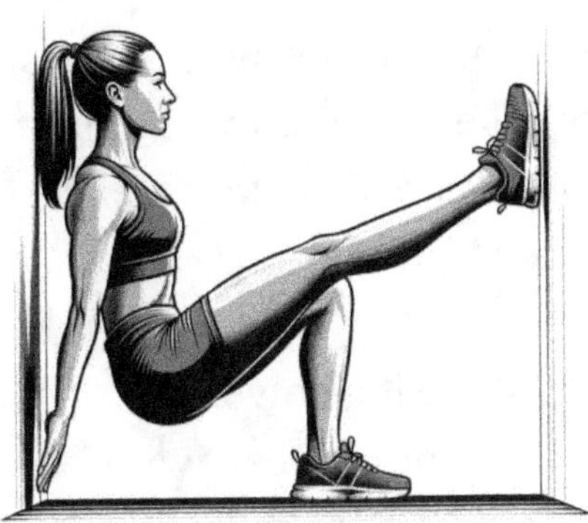

Wall Sit Leg Lifts combine the stability and endurance challenge of a wall sit with the added intensity of leg lifts. This exercise is designed to strengthen the quadriceps, hamstrings, and core muscles, while also enhancing balance and muscular endurance. It's an excellent workout for those looking to increase lower body strength and stamina.

Instructions for Wall Sit Leg Lifts

1. Starting Position: Stand with your back against a wall. Walk your feet forward while sliding down the wall, bending your knees to a 90-degree angle. Your thighs should be parallel to the floor, and your back flat against the wall.

2. Movement: Once in the wall sit position, slowly lift one leg off the ground, extending it straight out in front of you. Keep your foot flexed and hold the leg in the air for a few seconds.

3. Return and Repeat: Lower the leg back to the starting position and repeat with the other leg. Alternate between legs for each repetition.

4. Breathing: Breathe in as you lift your leg and exhale as you lower it back down. Keep your breathing steady and controlled.

5. Posture: Ensure your back remains flat against the wall throughout the exercise. Engage your core to maintain balance and stability.

Number of Sets and Repetitions

☐ - Beginners: Start with 2 sets of 5 to 8 lifts per leg. Focus on maintaining proper form and balance.

☐ - Intermediate: Perform 3 sets of 10 to 12 lifts per leg.

☐ - Advanced: Increase the challenge by holding each lift for a longer duration or adding more sets.

Wall Sit Leg Lifts are a challenging exercise that targets multiple muscle groups simultaneously. They are especially beneficial for those looking to enhance their lower body strength and improve muscular endurance. Remember to perform the exercise at a controlled pace and focus on maintaining proper posture throughout.

Wall Plank Holds

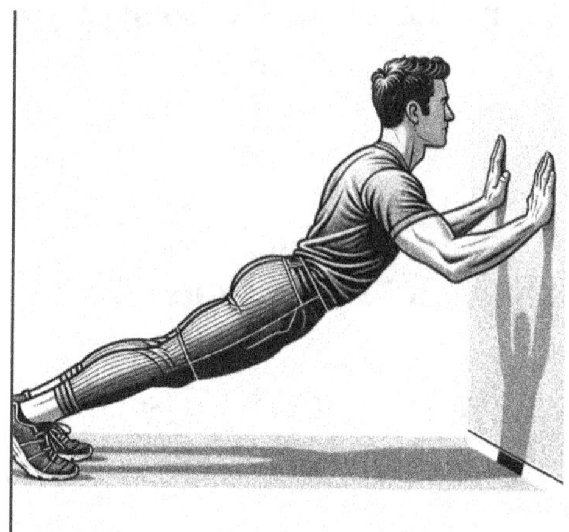

Wall Plank Holds are an excellent variation of the traditional floor plank that target the core muscles, including the abdominals, back, and shoulders. This exercise is beneficial for improving core stability, posture, and overall strength. The wall provides added support, making it a suitable option for individuals at various fitness levels or those who are building up to a full floor plank.

Instructions for Wall Plank Holds

1. Starting Position: Stand facing the wall at arm's length. Place your forearms on the wall at shoulder height, with elbows bent at a 90-degree angle.

2. Movement: Step back with your feet until your body forms a straight line from your head to your heels. Your body should be inclined to the wall at an angle.

3. Hold: Engage your core, squeezing your glutes and thighs to keep your body straight. Ensure your neck is in a neutral position, aligned with your spine.

4. Breathing: Maintain a steady breathing pattern. Inhale and exhale slowly, focusing on keeping your core engaged throughout the hold.

5. Posture: Keep your body as straight as possible, avoiding any sagging in your lower back or hiking of your hips.

Number of Sets and Repetitions

- ☐ - Beginners: Start with 2 to 3 sets of 20 to 30 seconds. Focus on maintaining proper form and alignment.
- ☐ - Intermediate: Aim for 3 sets of 45 seconds to 1 minute.

☐ - Advanced: Increase the duration or add variations, such as lifting one leg or one arm at a time. Try holding for longer than 1 minute or performing multiple sets.

Wall Plank Holds are a versatile and effective exercise for strengthening the core and enhancing stability. They are particularly beneficial for those working on their core strength or seeking a low-impact alternative to traditional planks. Remember to keep your movements controlled and focus on maintaining a strong, stable posture throughout the exercise.

Wall Mountain Climbers

Wall Mountain Climbers are a dynamic, high-intensity exercise that combines the benefits of cardiovascular training with core strengthening. This exercise is a variation of the traditional floor mountain climbers, with the wall adding an element of stability and reducing the impact on the wrists and shoulders. It's an excellent workout for increasing heart rate, burning calories, and engaging multiple muscle groups.

Instructions for Wall Mountain Climbers

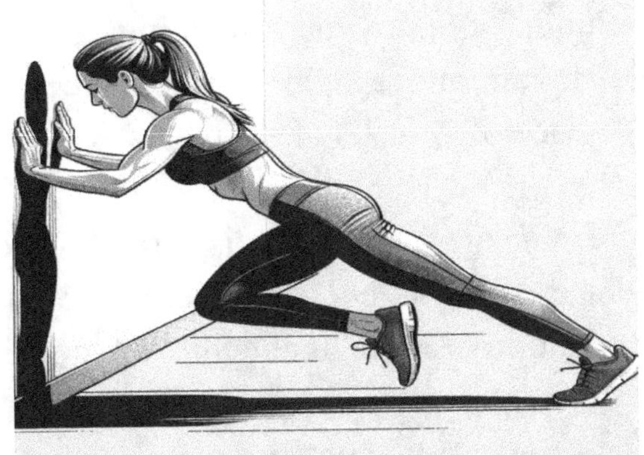

1. Starting Position: Stand facing the wall. Place your hands on the wall at shoulder height, about arm's length away. Step back so that your body forms an inclined plank position, with your feet hip-width apart.

2. Movement: Start by drawing one knee towards your chest, while keeping the other leg extended behind you. Quickly switch legs, bringing the other knee forward and extending the first leg back.

3. Rhythm: Maintain a fast pace, alternating legs quickly as if you're running in place against the wall. The movement should be fluid and continuous.

4. Breathing: Keep your breathing steady and rhythmic. Inhale and exhale in quick succession to match the pace of your leg movements.

5. Posture: Ensure your back is straight and your core is engaged throughout the exercise. Your body should remain in a stable, inclined plank position.

Number of Sets and Repetitions

- □ - Beginners: Start with 2 sets of 20 to 30 seconds each. Focus on maintaining form and building endurance.
- □ - Intermediate: Perform 3 sets of 30 to 45 seconds each, increasing the speed as you get more comfortable.
- □ - Advanced: Challenge yourself with longer durations or more sets, aiming for 3 to 5 sets of 1 minute or more.

Wall Mountain Climbers are a versatile and effective exercise for those looking to enhance their cardiovascular fitness and core strength. They are especially beneficial for anyone looking for a high-energy, low-impact workout. Remember to keep the movements controlled and focus on maintaining a strong, stable posture throughout the exercise.

Standing Wall Oblique Twists

Standing Wall Oblique Twists are a dynamic exercise targeting the oblique muscles, which are crucial for core strength, rotational movements, and overall stability. This exercise involves a twisting motion that engages the oblique muscles, providing an effective workout for toning the waistline and enhancing core stability. It's a great addition to any fitness routine aimed at developing a strong and defined midsection.

Instructions for Standing Wall Oblique Twists

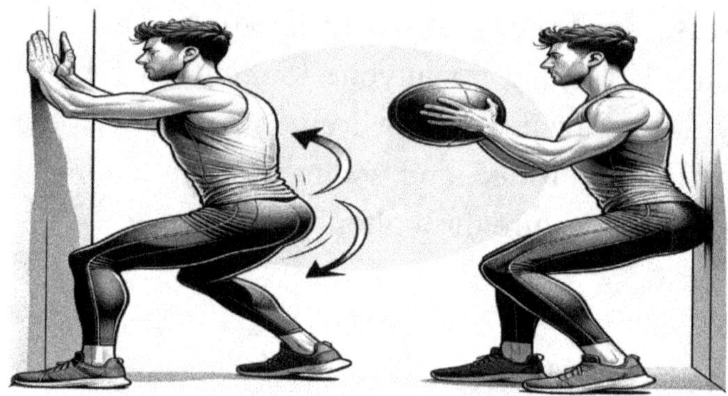

1. Starting Position: Stand sideways to the wall, about an arm's length away. Hold a medicine ball or a similar weighted object with both hands in front of you at chest height.

2. Movement: Keeping your hips and legs stationary, twist your torso to bring the ball towards the wall gently. Touch the wall with the ball, applying slight pressure.

3. Return Movement: Rotate your torso in the opposite direction, moving the ball across your body while maintaining your stance.

4. Breathing: Inhale as you twist to the wall, and exhale as you bring the ball across your body.

5. Posture: Keep your back straight and your core engaged throughout the exercise. The movement should come from your waist, not your hips or legs.

Number of Sets and Repetitions

- ☐ - Beginners: Start with 2 sets of 10 to 12 twists on each side. Focus on form and the engagement of your oblique muscles.
- ☐ - Intermediate: Perform 3 sets of 15 to 20 twists per side.
- ☐ - Advanced: Increase the challenge by using a heavier medicine ball or increasing the number of sets and repetitions.

Standing Wall Oblique Twists are an excellent exercise for those aiming to strengthen and define their oblique muscles. The controlled twisting motion not only helps tone the waistline but also enhances functional movements that involve rotation. Remember to perform the exercise with control, focusing on engaging your core and maintaining proper alignment throughout the movement.

Wall Supported Leg Circles

Wall Supported Leg Circles are an excellent exercise for improving flexibility, leg strength, and hip mobility. This exercise involves circular movements of the leg while using the wall for support, making it a fantastic choice for those focusing on controlled, precise leg movements. It's particularly beneficial for enhancing joint mobility and muscle control in the hips and legs.

Instructions for Wall Supported Leg Circles

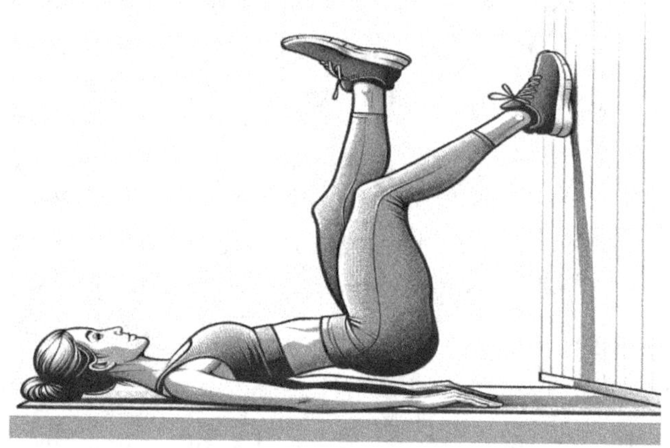

1. Starting Position: Lie on your back on a mat, facing the wall. Lift your legs and press them against the wall, keeping them straight. Your body and legs should form a 90-degree angle.

2. Movement: Keeping one leg pressed against the wall, slowly move the other leg in a circular motion. The movement should be controlled and originate from the hip.

3. Direction and Range: Perform the circles both clockwise and counterclockwise. The range of motion depends on your flexibility – start small and gradually increase.

4. Switch Legs: After completing the set with one leg, switch to the other leg and repeat the exercise.

5. Breathing: Inhale as you start the circle, and exhale as you complete it. Keep your breathing steady and controlled.

6. Posture: Ensure your back remains flat on the mat, and your core is engaged throughout the exercise.

Number of Sets and Repetitions

- ☐ - Beginners: Start with 2 sets of 5 circles in each direction for each leg.

- ☐ - Intermediate: Perform 3 sets of 8 to 10 circles in each direction per leg.
- ☐ - Advanced: Increase the size of the circles or the number of repetitions for a more challenging workout.

Wall Supported Leg Circles are a fantastic way to enhance the flexibility and strength of your lower body, especially around the hips. They're also beneficial for improving your control over leg movements, which is valuable in various physical activities and sports. Remember to perform the exercise with control and within your range of motion to prevent any strain.

Inverted Wall Crunches

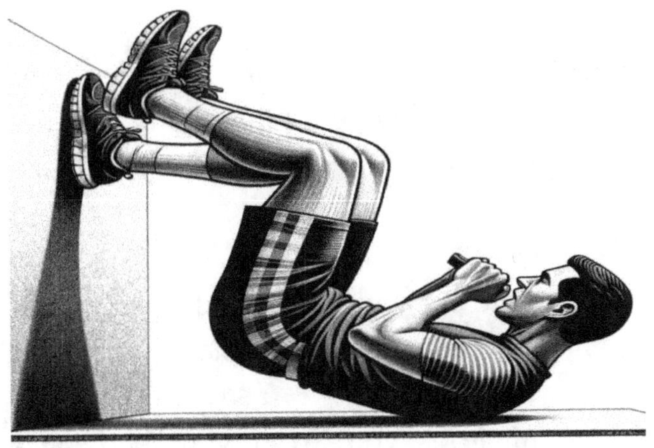

Inverted Wall Crunches are a unique variation of the traditional crunch exercise, utilizing a wall to increase the intensity and effectiveness of the workout. This exercise specifically targets the abdominal muscles, enhancing core strength and stability. It's an excellent choice for those looking to add a challenging twist to their core workouts.

Instructions for Inverted Wall Crunches

1. Starting Position: Lie on your back on a mat, placing your hips close to the wall. Raise your legs

and press them against the wall, forming a 90-degree angle at both your hips and knees.

2. Movement: Engage your core muscles and perform a crunch by lifting your upper body towards your knees. Keep your neck relaxed and your gaze upwards.

3. Return: Slowly lower your upper body back to the mat, maintaining control throughout the movement.

4. Breathing: Inhale as you lower your body and exhale as you lift into the crunch.

5. Posture: Ensure that your lower back remains in contact with the mat throughout the exercise to avoid any strain.

Number of Sets and Repetitions

- □ - Beginners: Start with 2 sets of 8 to 10 repetitions. Focus on engaging your core and maintaining proper form.
- □ - Intermediate: Perform 3 sets of 12 to 15 repetitions.

☐ - Advanced: Increase the intensity by holding the crunch position for a few seconds or adding more sets and repetitions.

Inverted Wall Crunches are a powerful exercise for strengthening the abdominal muscles and enhancing core stability. They offer a more challenging approach to traditional crunches, making them ideal for those looking to intensify their core workouts. Remember to perform the exercise with control, focusing on engaging your abdominal muscles throughout the movement.

Wall Bridge Lifts

Wall Bridge Lifts are an effective exercise for strengthening the glutes, hamstrings, and core. This exercise is a variation of the traditional bridge, using a wall to add stability and intensity. It's excellent for improving lower body strength, enhancing pelvic stability, and can be particularly beneficial for those looking to alleviate lower back pain.

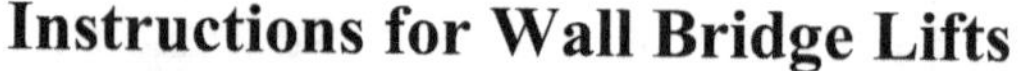

Instructions for Wall Bridge Lifts

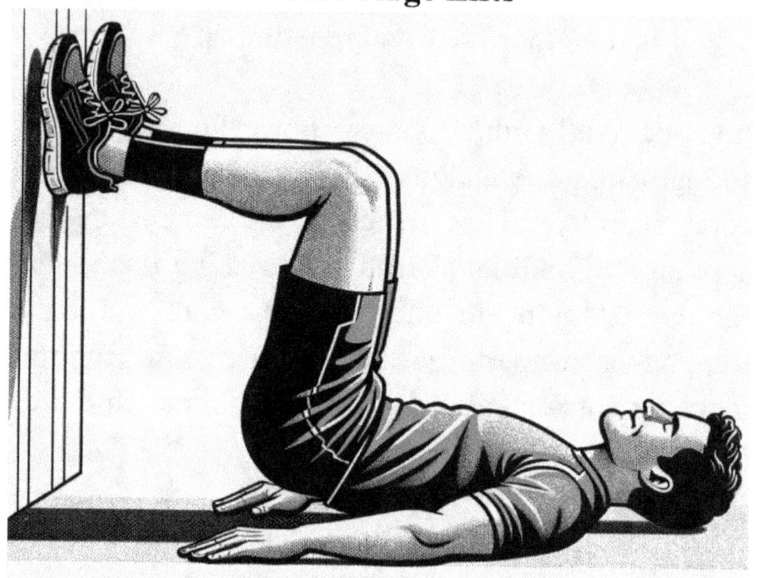

1. Starting Position: Lie on your back with your arms flat on the ground for support. Place your feet flat against the wall, knees bent so that your thighs and calves form a 90-degree angle.

2. Movement: Engage your core and glutes to lift your hips off the ground, forming a straight line from your shoulders to your knees. Keep your feet pressed against the wall.

3. Hold and Return: Hold the lifted position for a few seconds, then slowly lower your hips back down to the starting position.

4. Breathing: Inhale as you lower your hips and exhale as you lift them upwards.

5. Posture: Ensure that your movements are controlled and your spine remains in a neutral position throughout the exercise.

Number of Sets and Repetitions

- □ - Beginners: Start with 2 sets of 8 to 10 repetitions. Focus on engaging your glutes and maintaining control.
- □ - Intermediate: Perform 3 sets of 12 to 15 repetitions.
- □ - Advanced: Increase the challenge by holding the lifted position for a longer duration or adding more sets and repetitions.

Wall Bridge Lifts are a fantastic exercise for targeting the lower body and core. They are especially useful for those looking to strengthen their glutes and hamstrings while also working on their core stability. Remember to perform the exercise with control, focusing on maintaining proper form and alignment throughout the movement.

Side Wall Planks with Rotation

Side Wall Planks with Rotation are an advanced variation of the classic side plank exercise, adding a rotational movement to engage the core and oblique muscles further. This exercise combines core stabilization with dynamic movement, enhancing balance, strength, and flexibility. It's particularly effective for those looking to challenge their core muscles and improve overall body control.

Instructions for Side Wall Planks with Rotation

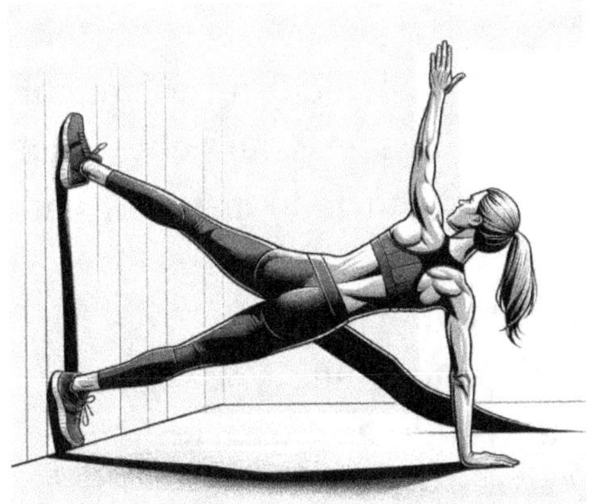

1. Starting Position: Begin in a side plank position with your feet against the wall. Place your forearm on the ground, ensuring it's directly below your shoulder. Extend your other arm towards the ceiling.

2. Movement: Keeping your feet against the wall for support, rotate your torso towards the ground and reach under your body with your extended arm.

3. Rotation and Return: Rotate back to the starting position, extending your arm back towards the ceiling. This completes one repetition.

4. Breathing: Inhale as you rotate and reach under your body, and exhale as you return to the starting position.

5. Posture: Keep your body in a straight line from head to feet. Engage your core and obliques throughout the movement to maintain stability.

Visual Representation
Here's an image to guide you through the proper form for Side Wall Planks with Rotation:

Number of Sets and Repetitions

- Beginners: Start with 2 sets of 5 to 8 repetitions on each side. Focus on maintaining form and control.
- Intermediate: Perform 3 sets of 10 to 12 repetitions on each side.
- Advanced: Increase the challenge by holding the rotation for a few seconds or adding more sets and repetitions.

Side Wall Planks with Rotation are a challenging yet rewarding exercise for enhancing core strength and stability. They require focus and control, making them an excellent addition to any workout routine aimed at improving core performance and stability. Remember to perform the exercise within your comfort level and focus on maintaining proper alignment throughout the movement.

Wall Reverse Crunches

Wall Reverse Crunches are a powerful exercise for targeting the lower abdominal muscles. This exercise adds a unique twist to the traditional reverse crunch by incorporating a wall for added resistance and control. It's especially effective for those looking to strengthen their core, improve pelvic control, and target the often challenging lower abs.

Instructions for Wall Reverse Crunches

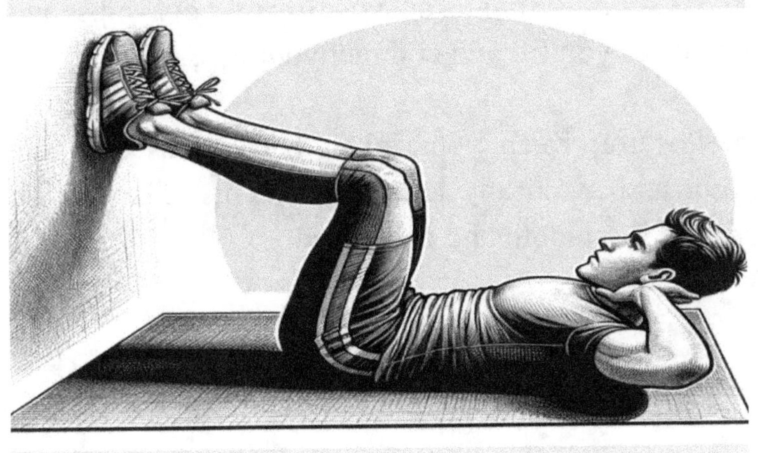

1. Starting Position: Lie on your back on a mat, with your arms flat on the ground or on your neck for stability. Position your legs up with your feet flat against the wall, forming a 90-degree angle at both your hips and knees.

2. Movement: Engage your core muscles and lift your hips off the ground, bringing your knees towards your chest. Your feet should slide down the wall as you perform the movement.

3. Return: Slowly lower your hips back to the starting position, controlling the movement to maintain engagement in your abdominal muscles.

4. Breathing: Inhale as you lower your hips and exhale as you lift and contract your abs.

5. Posture: Keep your lower back pressed to the floor and avoid any jerky movements. The motion should be smooth and controlled.

Number of Sets and Repetitions

- □ - Beginners: Start with 2 sets of 8 to 10 repetitions. Focus on engaging your lower abs and maintaining control.
- □ - Intermediate: Perform 3 sets of 12 to 15 repetitions.
- □ - Advanced: Increase the challenge by holding the lifted position for a few seconds or adding more sets and repetitions.

Wall Reverse Crunches are an excellent exercise for deep core engagement and targeting the lower abs. They provide a controlled and effective way to strengthen the core, crucial for overall stability and strength. Remember to perform the exercise with control, focusing on engaging your abdominal muscles throughout the movement.

Wall V-Sits

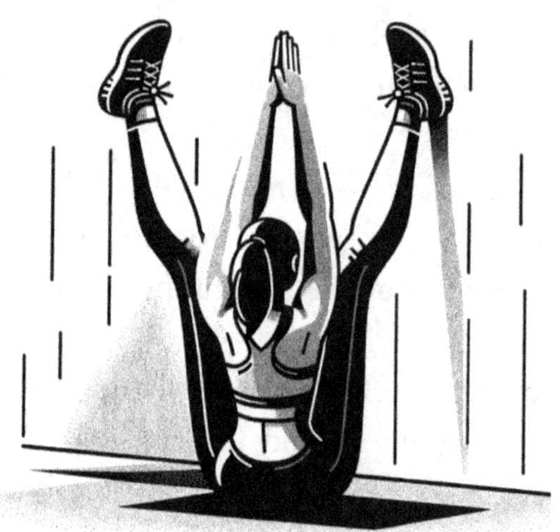

Wall V-Sits are a challenging core exercise that enhances strength, balance, and flexibility. This exercise is a variation of the traditional V-Sit, using the wall as a support for the back. It's particularly effective for engaging the abdominal muscles, improving posture, and enhancing core stability.

Instructions for Wall V-Sits

1. Starting Position: Sit on the floor with your back against the wall. Keep your legs together and straight in front of you, and arms by your sides.

2. Movement: Lift your legs off the floor, keeping them straight. Lean back slightly against the wall for support as you raise your legs.

3. Forming the 'V' Shape: Extend your arms towards your raised legs, forming a 'V' shape with your body. Engage your core to maintain balance.

4. Hold and Return: Hold the position for a few seconds, then slowly lower your legs and return to the starting position.

5. Breathing: Inhale as you prepare to lift your legs, and exhale as you raise them into the V-Sit position.

6. Posture: Ensure your movements are controlled and your back remains straight throughout the exercise.

Number of Sets and Repetitions

- □ - Beginners: Start with 2 sets of 5 to 8 repetitions. Focus on maintaining form and control.

- ☐ - Intermediate: Perform 3 sets of 10 to 12 repetitions.
- ☐ - Advanced: Increase the difficulty by holding the V-Sit position longer or adding more sets and repetitions.

Wall V-Sits are an excellent exercise for those looking to strengthen their core muscles and improve overall stability. The use of the wall for support allows for focus on form and engagement of the correct muscles. Remember to perform the exercise within your comfort level and focus on maintaining proper alignment and control throughout the movement.

CHAPTER 5: FLEXIBILITY EXERCISES

Wall-Assisted Hamstring Stretch

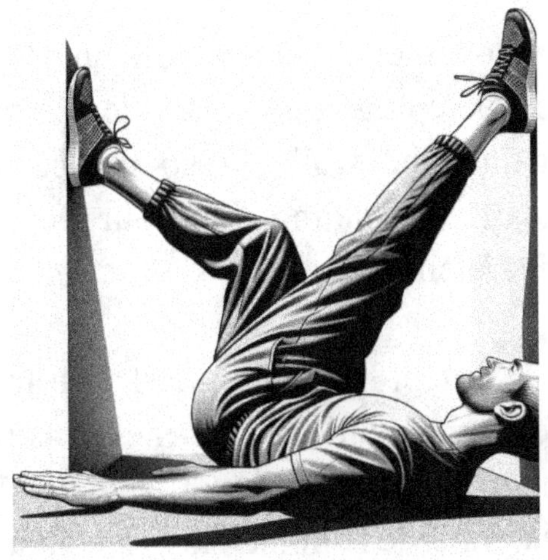

The Wall-Assisted Hamstring Stretch is an effective and gentle way to enhance flexibility in the hamstrings, crucial for a range of activities and overall leg health. Particularly within Wall Pilates, this stretch integrates the principles of controlled movement and alignment, making it an ideal choice for improving flexibility and reducing tension in the lower body.

Instructions for Wall-Assisted Hamstring Stretch

1. Starting Position: Lie on your back on a mat, close to a wall. Lift your legs and place them straight against the wall, forming a 90-degree angle with your body.

2. Stretch Movement: Gently pull one leg towards your chest, keeping the other leg straight and pressed against the wall. Grasp the back of your thigh or calf, depending on your flexibility, to deepen the stretch.

3. Hold the Stretch: Maintain the stretch for 20 to 30 seconds, feeling a gentle pull in the hamstring of the extended leg. Your back should remain flat on the mat, and the other leg should stay in contact with the wall.

4. Switching Legs: Carefully return the leg to the wall and repeat the stretch with the other leg.

5. Breathing: Breathe deeply and steadily during the stretch. Inhale as you prepare for the stretch and exhale as you gently deepen it.

6. Posture: Keep your hips squared and aligned. Your upper body should remain relaxed on the mat.

Number of Sets and Repetitions

- ☐ - Frequency: This stretch can be performed daily, especially after leg-intensive workouts or periods of prolonged sitting.
- ☐ - Duration: Hold each stretch for 20 to 30 seconds per leg. Repeat 2 to 3 times on each side for maximum benefit.

The Wall-Assisted Hamstring Stretch is excellent for increasing leg flexibility, which is vital for a range of physical activities and overall mobility. It's a simple yet effective way to alleviate tightness in the hamstrings and can be easily incorporated into your regular fitness or Pilates routine. Remember to perform the stretch gently and within your comfort range to avoid any strain.

Standing Wall Calf Stretch

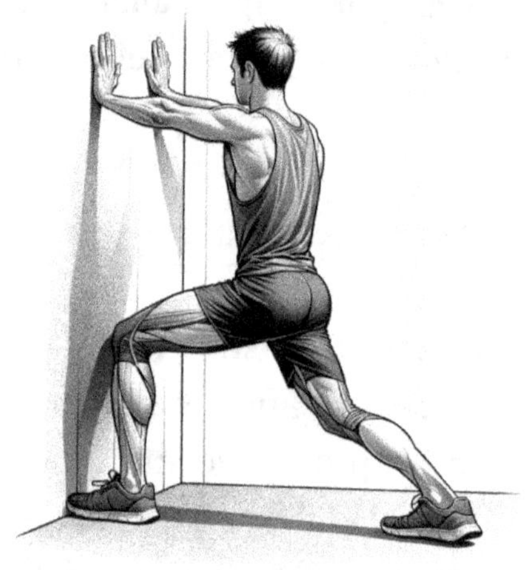

The Standing Wall Calf Stretch is a simple yet highly effective exercise for loosening tight calf muscles, which are crucial for various activities like walking, running, and jumping. This stretch is particularly beneficial for people who spend a lot of time on their feet or those who engage in sports. It helps to improve flexibility in the calf muscles and can prevent injuries related to muscle tightness.

Instructions for Standing Wall Calf Stretch

Pg. 118

1. Starting Position: Stand facing a wall. Place your hands on the wall at shoulder height for support.

2. Movement: Step one leg back, keeping your heel pressed to the floor. The other leg should be bent forward. Ensure both feet are pointing straight ahead.

3. Stretch: Lean into the wall, keeping your back leg straight, to deepen the stretch in the calf muscle. You should feel a gentle pull in the lower part of your extended leg.

4. Hold and Switch: Hold the stretch for about 20 to 30 seconds, then switch legs and repeat.

5. Breathing: Breathe deeply and steadily during the stretch. Exhale as you deepen the stretch to enhance muscle relaxation.

6. Posture: Keep your hips square and facing the wall. Ensure the heel of your extended leg remains in contact with the floor throughout the stretch.

Number of Sets and Repetitions

☐ - Frequency: This stretch can be performed daily, especially after activities that strain the calf muscles.

☐ - Duration: Hold each stretch for 20 to 30 seconds per leg. Repeat 2 to 3 times on each side for optimal results.

The Standing Wall Calf Stretch is an excellent way to maintain calf muscle flexibility, which is essential for mobility and injury prevention. It's a straightforward and effective stretch that can be easily incorporated into any daily routine or workout regimen. Remember to perform the stretch gently and within a comfortable range to avoid overstretching.

Wall Shoulder Opener Stretch

The Wall Shoulder Opener Stretch is an effective exercise for loosening tight shoulder and chest muscles. This stretch is particularly beneficial for individuals who spend long hours at a desk or engaging in activities that lead to poor posture. It helps to improve shoulder flexibility, open up the chest, and can significantly enhance upper body mobility.

Instructions for Wall Shoulder Opener Stretch

1. Starting Position: Stand sideways next to a wall. Extend the arm closest to the wall and place it flat against the wall at shoulder height. Your palm should be flat and fingers pointing away from your body.

2. Movement: Gently turn your body away from the wall, focusing on stretching the shoulder and chest muscles of the extended arm. Keep your arm straight throughout the stretch.

3. Hold and Release: Hold the stretch for about 20 to 30 seconds, feeling a gentle opening in your shoulder and chest. Release and switch sides to repeat the stretch with the other arm.

4. Breathing: Breathe deeply and steadily during the stretch. Exhale as you deepen the stretch to enhance muscle relaxation.

5. Posture: Keep your body upright and avoid overstretching. Controlled and seamless movement is required.

Number of Sets and Repetitions

- ☐ - Beginners: Start with 2 sets of 20 to 30 seconds per arm. Focus on a gentle stretch without straining.
- ☐ - Intermediate: Perform 3 sets, holding for up to 45 seconds per arm.
- ☐ - Advanced: Increase the duration or intensity by holding the stretch longer or incorporating gentle movement to deepen the stretch.

The Wall Shoulder Opener Stretch is an excellent exercise for releasing tension in the upper body and improving overall flexibility in the shoulders and chest. It's a simple and effective stretch that can be easily incorporated into any daily routine or workout regimen. Remember to perform the stretch gently and within a comfortable range to avoid overstretching.

Wall-Assisted Chest Stretch

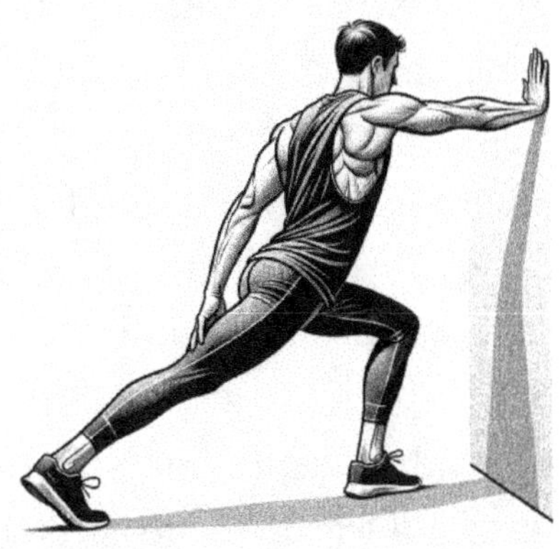

The Wall-Assisted Chest Stretch is a simple and effective exercise to open up and stretch the chest muscles. This stretch is particularly beneficial for individuals who spend a lot of time sitting or have activities that round the shoulders forward. It helps to alleviate tightness in the chest and shoulders, improving posture and upper body flexibility.

Instructions for Wall-Assisted Chest Stretch

1. Starting Position: Stand facing a wall. Extend one arm to the side and place your palm flat against the wall at shoulder height.

2. Movement: Gently turn your body away from the wall, keeping your arm extended. You should feel a stretch across the chest muscles of the extended arm.

3. Hold and Release: Hold the stretch for 20 to 30 seconds, then slowly return to the starting position. Switch arms and repeat the stretch.

4. Breathing: Breathe deeply and steadily during the stretch. Inhale as you prepare to stretch and exhale as you deepen the stretch.

5. Posture: Keep your body upright and avoid overstretching. Controlled and seamless movement is required.

Number of Sets and Repetitions

- ☐ - Beginners: Start with 2 sets of 20 to 30 seconds per arm. Focus on a gentle stretch without straining.
- ☐ - Intermediate: Perform 3 sets, holding for up to 45 seconds per arm.
- ☐ - Advanced: Increase the duration or intensity by holding the stretch longer or incorporating gentle movement to deepen the stretch.

The Wall-Assisted Chest Stretch is a great way to improve flexibility in the chest and shoulder area. It's a straightforward exercise that can be easily incorporated into any daily routine or workout regimen, helping to counteract the effects of poor posture and muscle tightness. Remember to perform the stretch gently and within a comfortable range to avoid overstretching.

Wall-Supported Side Stretch

The Wall-Supported Side Stretch is an excellent exercise for increasing flexibility and range of motion in the torso and lateral muscles. This stretch is beneficial for those who experience tightness in the sides of the body, often due to prolonged sitting or repetitive activities. It helps in lengthening the muscles along the sides of the body, improving posture and reducing tension.

Instructions for Wall-Supported Side Stretch

1. Starting Position: Stand sideways next to a wall. Place the hand closest to the wall on it for support, at about shoulder height.

2. Movement: Raise your other arm over your head and lean towards the wall, creating a deep stretch along the side of your torso. Ensure your hips stay aligned and don't push forward.

3. Hold and Release: Hold the stretch for 20 to 30 seconds, feeling a gentle elongation along your side. Gently return to the starting position and switch sides.

4. Breathing: Inhale deeply as you extend your arm, and exhale as you deepen the stretch.

5. Posture: Keep your spine long and avoid collapsing the torso. The movement should come from the waist.

Number of Sets and Repetitions

- ☐ - Beginners: Start with 2 sets of 20 to 30 seconds per side. Focus on a gentle stretch without straining.
- ☐ - Intermediate: Perform 3 sets of up to 45 seconds per side.
- ☐ - Advanced: Increase the duration or intensity by holding the stretch longer or incorporating gentle movement to deepen the stretch.

The Wall-Supported Side Stretch is an effective way to relieve tightness and improve flexibility in the sides of the torso. It's a simple exercise that can be easily incorporated into any daily routine or workout regimen, helping to maintain good posture and overall body flexibility. Remember to perform the stretch gently and within a comfortable range to avoid overstretching.

<u>Wall-Assisted Triceps Stretch</u>

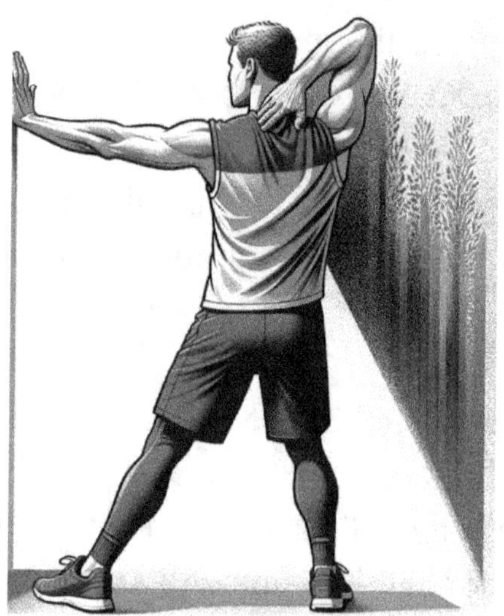

The Wall-Assisted Triceps Stretch is a targeted exercise designed to stretch and relieve tension in the triceps muscles. This stretch is particularly useful for those engaged in activities that heavily involve the arms and shoulders. It helps in improving the flexibility of the upper arms, essential for a full range of motion and injury prevention.

Instructions for Wall-Assisted Triceps Stretch

1. Starting Position: Stand with your back to a wall. Reach one arm overhead and bend it so that your

hand reaches down the middle of your back, with your elbow pointing upwards.

2. Movement: Using the wall for balance and support, gently press your bent elbow with your other hand to deepen the stretch. You should feel a gentle pull along the tricep of the bent arm.

3. Hold and Switch: Hold the stretch for about 20 to 30 seconds, then release and switch arms, repeating the stretch.

4. Breathing: Inhale as you reach up and exhale as you deepen the stretch. Breathe deeply to facilitate muscle relaxation.

5. Posture: Keep your spine straight and avoid leaning forward or backward.

Number of Sets and Repetitions

- ☐ - Beginners: Start with 2 sets of 20 to 30 seconds per arm. Focus on a gentle stretch without straining.

- ☐ - Intermediate: Perform 2 to 3 sets of up to 45 seconds per arm.
- ☐ - Advanced: Increase the duration or intensity by holding the stretch longer or incorporating gentle movement to deepen the stretch.

The Wall-Assisted Triceps Stretch is an effective way to increase flexibility in the upper arms and relieve tightness. It's a straightforward exercise that can be easily incorporated into any daily routine or workout regimen, helping to maintain good arm health and prevent stiffness. Remember to perform the stretch gently and within a comfortable range to avoid overstretching.

Wall-Assisted Hip Flexor Stretch

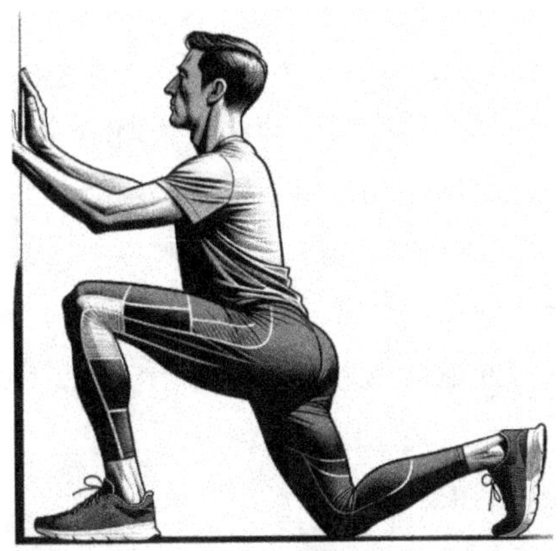

The Wall-Assisted Hip Flexor Stretch is a highly effective exercise designed to stretch and relieve tightness in the hip flexor muscles. This stretch is particularly valuable for individuals who sit for prolonged periods or engage in activities with repetitive leg movements. It aids in improving flexibility in the hip area and can help prevent lower back pain and improve posture.

Instructions for Wall-Assisted Hip Flexor Stretch

1. Starting Position: Kneel down and face away from the wall. Place the knee of one leg on the

ground close to the wall, and the foot of your other leg in front, forming a lunge position.

2. Movement: Lean your back knee against the wall for added stretch. Gently push your hips forward to deepen the stretch in the hip flexors of the back leg.

3. Hold and Switch: Hold the stretch for 20 to 30 seconds, feeling a deep stretch in the front of your hip. Gently release and switch to the other leg, repeating the stretch.

4. Breathing: Inhale as you set up the position, and exhale as you deepen the stretch. Breathe deeply to enhance muscle relaxation.

5. Posture: Keep your upper body upright, and avoid arching your lower back excessively.

Number of Sets and Repetitions

- ☐ - Beginners: Start with 2 sets of 20 to 30 seconds per leg. Focus on a gentle stretch without straining.

☐ - Intermediate: Perform 2 to 3 sets of up to 45 seconds per leg.

☐ - Advanced: Increase the duration or intensity by holding the stretch longer or incorporating gentle movements to deepen the stretch.

The Wall-Assisted Hip Flexor Stretch is an excellent way to alleviate tightness in the hip flexors and improve lower body flexibility. It's a simple exercise that can be easily incorporated into any daily routine or workout regimen, helping to maintain hip health and prevent stiffness. Remember to perform the stretch gently and within a comfortable range to avoid overstretching.

Wall Supported Forward Bend

The Wall Supported Forward Bend is a deeply stretching exercise that targets the hamstrings, lower back, and calves. This stretch is particularly beneficial for those who experience tightness in these areas, whether due to prolonged sitting, intense physical activity, or natural stiffness. The wall provides support and allows for a more controlled and effective stretch.

Instructions for Wall Supported Forward Bend

1. Starting Position: Stand with your back against a wall. Your feet should be hip-width apart and parallel.

2. Movement: Slowly bend forward at the hips while keeping your back straight. Reach towards your toes. Your hands can touch the floor, your ankles, or rest on your shins, depending on your flexibility.

3. Hold and Release: Hold the forward bend for 20 to 30 seconds, feeling a stretch in your hamstrings and lower back. Keep your legs straight but avoid locking your knees.

4. Breathing: Inhale as you stand upright, and exhale as you bend forward. Breathe deeply to facilitate muscle relaxation.

5. Posture: Ensure your back remains straight as you fold forward. The wall will help maintain alignment.

Number of Sets and Repetitions

- □ - Beginners: Start with 2 sets of 20 to 30 seconds. Focus on feeling a gentle stretch without straining.
- □ - Intermediate: Perform 2 to 3 sets of up to 45 seconds.
- □ - Advanced: Increase the duration or intensity by holding the stretch longer or incorporating gentle movements to deepen the stretch.

The Wall Supported Forward Bend is an excellent way to improve flexibility in the lower body and alleviate tightness in the hamstrings and lower back. It's a simple exercise that can be easily incorporated into any daily routine or workout regimen, helping to maintain good flexibility and prevent stiffness. Remember to perform the stretch gently and within a comfortable range to avoid overstretching.

Wall-Assisted Spinal Twist

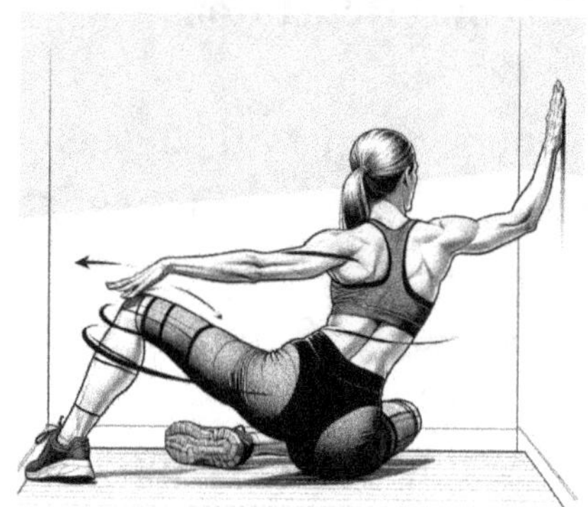

The Wall-Assisted Spinal Twist is a rejuvenating stretch that targets the spine, promoting flexibility and relieving tension in the back. It is excellent for decompressing the spine after long periods of sitting or as part of a cooldown in a workout routine. This twist aids in loosening up the back muscles and improving spinal mobility, contributing to overall back health.

Instructions for Wall-Assisted Spinal Twist

1. Starting Position: Sit on the floor with your back against the wall. Your legs can be extended in front of you or with one leg bent for comfort.

2. Movement: Twist your torso to one side. Extend the arm on the side you're twisting towards along the wall for support, while your other arm crosses over to your opposite knee to deepen the twist.

3. Hold and Switch: Maintain the twisted position for about 20 to 30 seconds, experiencing a gentle stretch along your spine and back. Slowly return to the center and repeat on the other side.

4. Breathing: Inhale deeply as you sit upright, and exhale as you twist. Steady breathing helps deepen the stretch and relax the muscles.

5. Posture: Keep your spine straight and long during the twist. Avoid slumping or collapsing your shoulders.

Number of Sets and Repetitions

- ☐ - Beginners: Start with 2 sets of 20 to 30 seconds per side. Focus on a gentle stretch without overstraining.
- ☐ - Intermediate: Perform 2 to 3 sets of up to 45 seconds per side.

☐ - Advanced: Increase the duration or intensity by holding the stretch longer or incorporating gentle movements to deepen the stretch.

The Wall-Assisted Spinal Twist is a beneficial exercise for enhancing spinal flexibility and relieving tension in the back muscles. It's a simple, effective stretch that can be incorporated into any daily routine or workout regimen to maintain a healthy and supple spine. Remember to perform the stretch gently and within a comfortable range to avoid overstretching.

Wall-Assisted Quadriceps Stretch

The Wall-Assisted Quadriceps Stretch is an excellent exercise for loosening tight quadriceps, the muscle group at the front of the thigh. This stretch is especially beneficial for individuals who engage in running, biking, or any activity that heavily involves the legs. It helps in improving flexibility in the thigh area, reducing the risk of injury, and aiding in muscle recovery.

Instructions for Wall-Assisted Quadriceps Stretch

1. Starting Position: Stand facing away from the wall. Use one hand to rest on the wall for balance.

2. Movement: Bend one leg behind you and hold your ankle with the same-side hand. Ensure your knee is pointing downwards and not splayed out.

3. Stretch: Gently push your hips forward while pulling your ankle closer to your body. You should feel a stretch in the front of your thigh.

4. Hold and Switch: Maintain the stretch for 20 to 30 seconds, then gently release your leg and switch to the other side.

5. Breathing: Inhale as you set up the position, and exhale as you deepen the stretch.

6. Posture: Keep your body upright and your standing leg slightly bent to maintain balance.

Number of Sets and Repetitions

- ☐ - Beginners: Start with 2 sets of 20 to 30 seconds per leg. Focus on feeling a gentle stretch without straining.
- ☐ - Intermediate: Perform 2 to 3 sets of up to 45 seconds per leg.
- ☐ - Advanced: Increase the duration or intensity by holding the stretch longer or incorporating gentle movements to deepen the stretch.

The Wall-Assisted Quadriceps Stretch is a fantastic way to alleviate tightness in the thighs and improve lower body flexibility. It's a simple exercise that can be easily integrated into any daily routine or workout regimen, helping to maintain muscle health and prevent stiffness. Remember to perform the stretch gently and within a comfortable range to avoid overstretching.

CHAPTER 6: UPPER BODY EXERCISES

Wall Push-Ups

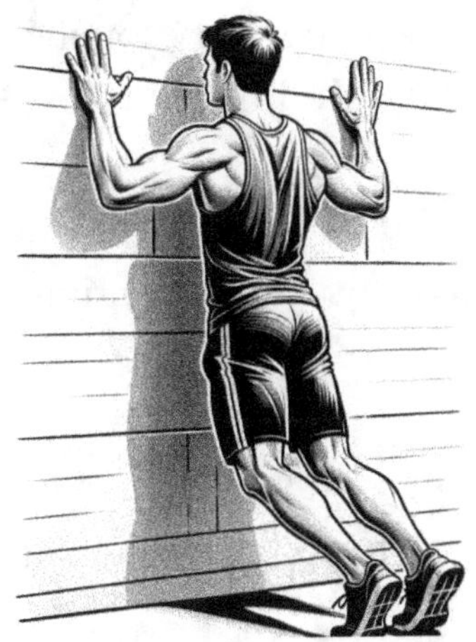

Wall Push-Ups are a fantastic exercise for beginners or those looking to strengthen their upper body without the intensity of traditional floor push-ups. This exercise targets the chest, shoulders, and triceps, and is also beneficial for improving overall upper body stability and strength. Wall Push-Ups are a great starting point for those new to fitness or as part of a rehabilitation program.

Instructions for Wall Push-Ups

1. Starting Position: Stand facing a wall, about an arm's length away. Place your hands on the wall at shoulder height and wider than shoulder-width apart.

2. Movement: Lean towards the wall, bending your elbows until your face nearly touches the wall. Keep your body in a straight line from head to heels.

3. Push Back: Push back to the starting position, extending your arms and engaging your chest and arm muscles.

4. Breathing: Inhale as you lean towards the wall and exhale as you push back to the starting position.

5. Posture: Maintain a straight back and engage your core throughout the exercise for stability.

Number of Sets and Repetitions

☐ - Beginners: Start with 2 sets of 8 to 10 repetitions. Focus on mastering the form and building strength.

☐ - Intermediate: Perform 3 sets of 12 to 15 repetitions.

☐ - Advanced: Increase the challenge by performing more sets or adding variations like single-leg wall push-ups.

Wall Push-Ups are an accessible and effective way to build upper body strength. They are versatile, can be done anywhere with a wall, and are suitable for all fitness levels. Remember to keep your movements controlled and focus on engaging your chest, arms, and core throughout the exercise.

Wall Tricep Dips

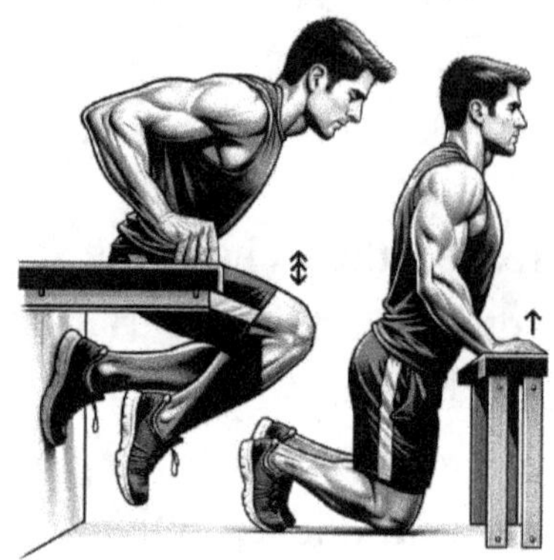

Wall Tricep Dips are an effective exercise for strengthening and toning the triceps muscles. They are a great alternative to traditional tricep dips and are particularly beneficial for those who may find floor or bench dips too challenging. This exercise can be easily modified to suit different fitness levels and is excellent for building upper arm strength.

Instructions for Wall Tricep Dips

1. Starting Position: Stand facing away from a low wall or a sturdy bench. Place your hands on the edge, shoulder-width apart.

2. Movement: Extend your legs forward, keeping your feet flat on the ground. Bend your elbows to a 90-degree angle and slowly lower your body.

3. Push Up: Push back up to the starting position by straightening your arms, focusing on engaging your triceps.

4. Breathing: Breathe in as you lower yourself and out as you raise yourself back up.

5. Posture: Keep your back close to the wall or bench throughout the exercise. Avoid letting your hips sag.

Number of Sets and Repetitions

- ☐ - Beginners: Start with 2 sets of 8 to 10 repetitions. Focus on maintaining proper form.
- ☐ - Intermediate: Perform 3 sets of 10 to 12 repetitions.
- ☐ - Advanced: Increase the challenge by adding more sets or elevating your feet to intensify the exercise.

Wall Tricep Dips are a versatile and effective way to target the triceps, making them a valuable addition to any upper body workout. Remember to keep your movements controlled and focus on engaging your triceps throughout the exercise.

Wall Arm Slides

Wall Arm Slides are an effective exercise for improving shoulder mobility and strengthening the muscles of the upper back and shoulders. This exercise is particularly beneficial for individuals who experience stiffness in the shoulder area or who spend long periods sitting at a desk. Wall Arm Slides help in promoting proper posture and can be a valuable addition to a shoulder rehabilitation program.

Instructions for Wall Arm Slides

1. Starting Position: Stand with your back against the wall. Raise your arms and bend your elbows at 90 degrees, placing your forearms and the backs of your hands against the wall.

2. Movement: Slide your arms up the wall, keeping your back, arms, and hands in contact with the wall throughout the movement. Extend as far as you comfortably can.

3. Return Movement: Slowly slide your arms back down to the starting position.

4. Breathing: Inhale as you slide your arms up and exhale as you return them to the starting position.

5. Posture: Keep your back flat against the wall and maintain the 90-degree bend in your elbows throughout the exercise.

Number of Sets and Repetitions

- ☐ - Beginners: Start with 2 sets of 8 to 10 slides. Focus on smooth movement and maintaining contact with the wall.
- ☐ - Intermediate: Perform 3 sets of 10 to 12 slides.
- ☐ - Advanced: Increase the challenge by adding more sets or holding at the top of the movement for a few seconds.

Wall Arm Slides are a great way to enhance shoulder mobility and strengthen the upper back and shoulder muscles. They are a low-impact exercise, making them suitable for people of all fitness levels. Remember to perform the exercise with control, focusing on keeping your arms and back in contact with the wall throughout the movement.

Wall Chest Squeezes

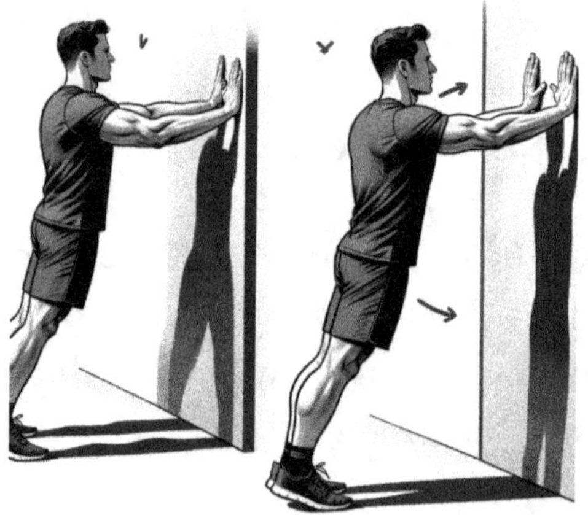

Wall Chest Squeezes are a simple yet effective exercise designed to strengthen and tone the chest muscles. This exercise is particularly beneficial for those who are looking for an alternative to traditional chest exercises like push-ups or bench presses. It's ideal for beginners or those who prefer low-impact exercises.

Instructions for Wall Chest Squeezes

1. Starting Position: Stand facing a wall. Extend your arms and place your palms flat against the wall at chest height.

2. Movement: Push into the wall, engaging your chest muscles as if you are trying to move the wall. Keep your arms straight and your body upright.

3. Release: Release the pressure slightly while maintaining contact with the wall, then push again.

4. Breathing: Inhale as you release the pressure and exhale as you push into the wall.

5. Posture: Ensure your body is aligned and your feet are planted firmly on the ground.

Number of Sets and Repetitions

☐ - Beginners: Start with 2 sets of 10 to 12 squeezes. Focus on maintaining constant pressure and form.

☐ - Intermediate: Increase to 3 sets of 15 squeezes.

☐ - Advanced: Add more sets or increase the duration of each squeeze for a greater challenge.

Wall Chest Squeezes are an excellent way to build strength in the chest muscles without the need for weights or equipment. This exercise can be easily incorporated into any fitness routine, making it a versatile choice for individuals of all fitness levels. Remember to perform the movement with control and focus on engaging your chest muscles throughout the exercise.

Wall Bicep Curls (Using Resistance Bands)

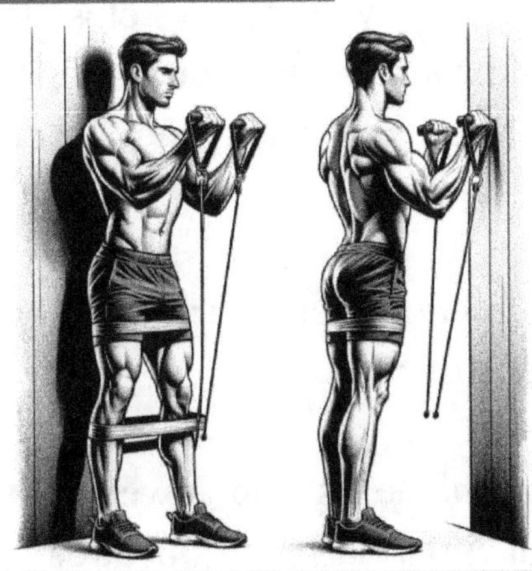

Wall Bicep Curls with resistance bands are an effective exercise for strengthening and toning the biceps. This variation, which includes the stability of a wall, is excellent for maintaining proper posture and alignment during the exercise. It's ideal for those who are looking to isolate their biceps without straining other parts of the body.

Instructions for Wall Bicep Curls (Using Resistance Bands)

1. Starting Position: Stand with your back against the wall. Place a resistance band under your feet and hold it with both hands.

2. Movement: With your elbows close to your body, bend your elbows and curl your hands towards your shoulders. Keep your back and head against the wall.

3. Return: Slowly lower your hands back down to the starting position.

4. Breathing: Inhale as you lower your hands and exhale as you curl your hands upwards.

5. Posture: Ensure your posture is straight, with your back and head against the wall throughout the exercise.

Number of Sets and Repetitions

- □ - Beginners: Start with 2 sets of 10 to 12 repetitions. Focus on form and controlled movement.

☐ - Intermediate: Perform 3 sets of 12 to 15 repetitions.

☐ - Advanced: Increase the resistance of the band or add more sets for a greater challenge.

Wall Bicep Curls with resistance bands are a great way to build bicep strength while ensuring proper form and posture. They are suitable for all fitness levels and can be easily modified by changing the resistance level of the band. Remember to keep your movements controlled and focus on engaging your biceps throughout the exercise.

Wall Plank Shoulder Taps

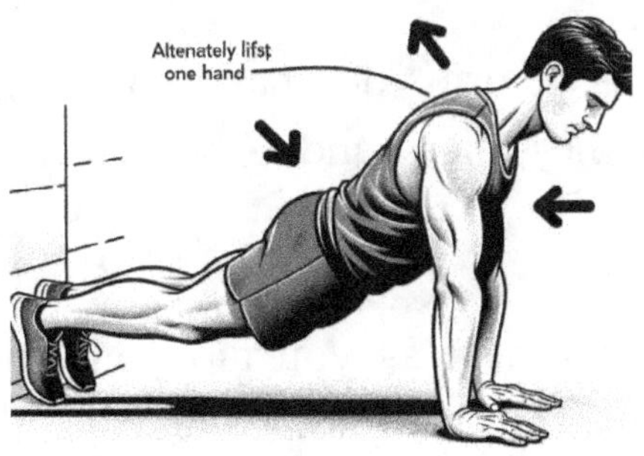

Wall Plank Shoulder Taps are an advanced variation of the traditional plank exercise, incorporating an element of balance and coordination. This exercise strengthens the core, shoulders, and arms, while also challenging stability and body control. It's an excellent choice for those looking to enhance their upper body and core strength with an added balance challenge.

Instructions for Wall Plank Shoulder Taps

1. Starting Position: Get into a plank position with your feet against the wall and hands on the ground, forming a straight line from head to heels.

2. Movement: Lift one hand to tap the opposite shoulder while maintaining the plank position. Keep your hips and shoulders as stable as possible.

3. Alternate: Return your hand to the ground and repeat with the other hand. Alternate taps between hands.

4. Breathing: Inhale as you tap your shoulder and exhale as you return your hand to the starting position.

5. Posture: Ensure your body remains in a straight line throughout the exercise. Avoid lifting your hips too high or letting them sag.

Number of Sets and Repetitions

- □ - Beginners: Start with 2 sets of 6 to 8 taps per hand. Focus on maintaining form and balance.
- □ - Intermediate: Perform 3 sets of 10 to 12 taps per hand.
- □ - Advanced: Increase the challenge by adding more sets or performing the taps more rapidly.

Wall Plank Shoulder Taps are a dynamic exercise that can significantly improve your core strength, stability, and upper body endurance. They are suitable for those who have mastered the basic plank and are looking to add variety to their core workouts. Remember to perform the exercise with control, focusing on keeping your plank position stable throughout the movement.

Wall Circles with Resistance Bands

Wall Circles with Resistance Bands are an innovative upper body exercise that combines the benefits of resistance training with dynamic movement to enhance shoulder mobility and strength. This exercise is excellent for those looking to improve their range of motion, shoulder stability, and muscle endurance in the arms and shoulders.

Instructions for Wall Circles with Resistance Bands

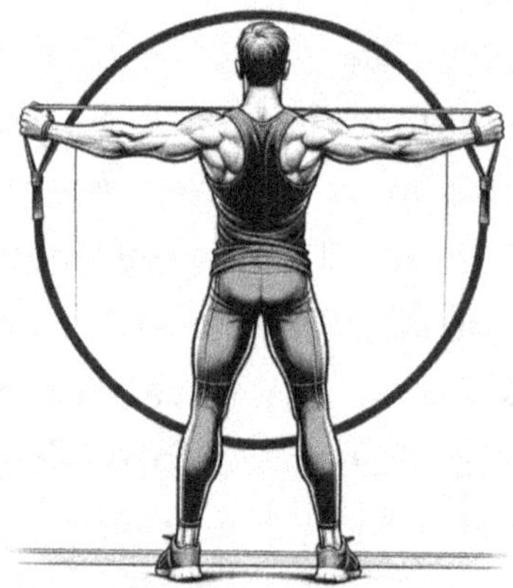

1. Starting Position: Stand facing a wall. Hold a resistance band with both hands, and extend your arms straight ahead at shoulder height.

2. Movement: Perform circular motions with your arms, keeping the resistance band taut. Ensure the movement is controlled and originates from the shoulders.

3. Direction and Range: Perform the circles both clockwise and counterclockwise. Adjust the range of motion to your comfort level.

4. Breathing: Inhale as you start the circle, and exhale as you complete it. Throughout the workout, keep the same breathing pattern.

5. Posture: Keep your back straight and your core engaged. Focus on moving your arms while keeping the rest of your body stable.

Number of Sets and Repetitions

- Beginners: Start with 2 sets of 6 to 8 circles in each direction.
- Intermediate: Increase to 3 sets of 10 to 12 circles in each direction.
- Advanced: Add more sets or increase the resistance of the band for a greater challenge.

Wall Circles with Resistance Bands are a versatile and effective exercise for improving shoulder health and building upper body strength. They can be easily incorporated into any fitness routine and are suitable for individuals of all fitness levels. Remember to perform the exercise with control, focusing on maintaining a steady range of motion and keeping the resistance band taut throughout the movement.

Wall Slide Shoulder Shrugs

Wall Slide Shoulder Shrugs are an excellent exercise for enhancing shoulder mobility and strengthening the upper trapezius muscles. This variation adds the stability of the wall to ensure proper posture and alignment throughout the exercise. It's particularly beneficial for those looking to relieve tension in the neck and upper back areas.

Instructions for Wall Slide Shoulder Shrugs

1. Starting Position: Stand with your back against the wall. Extend your arms straight up, with your palms facing forward. Your arms and back should remain in contact with the wall.

2. Movement: Perform shoulder shrugs by lifting your shoulders upwards towards your ears. Keep your arms extended and against the wall.

3. Return: Slowly lower your shoulders back down to the starting position.

4. Breathing: Inhale as you lift your shoulders and exhale as you lower them.

5. Posture: Ensure your back and arms remain in contact with the wall throughout the exercise to maintain alignment.

Number of Sets and Repetitions

- □ - Beginners: Start with 2 sets of 10 to 12 shrugs. Focus on smooth movement and maintaining contact with the wall.

☐ - Intermediate: Perform 3 sets of 12 to 15 shrugs.

☐ - Advanced: Increase the challenge by adding more sets or holding the shrug at the top position for a few seconds.

Wall Slide Shoulder Shrugs are a great way to improve shoulder health and reduce tension in the upper back and neck. They are a low-impact exercise, making them suitable for people of all fitness levels. Remember to perform the movement with control, focusing on keeping your arms and back in contact with the wall throughout the exercise.

Inverted Wall Rows

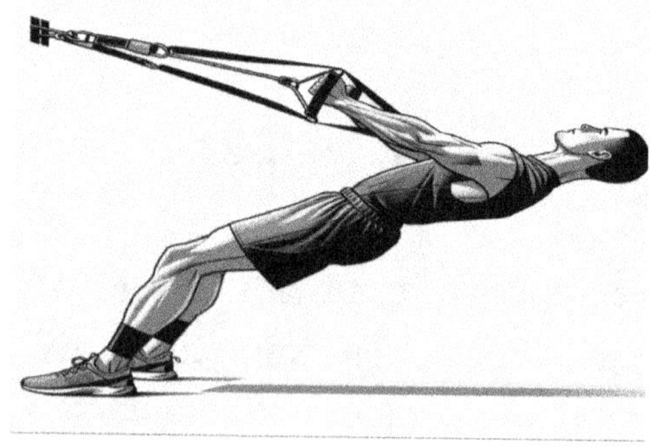

Inverted Wall Rows are a unique and effective exercise for strengthening the upper back and improving posture. This exercise uses a resistance band anchored above and the stability of a wall, making it a great alternative to traditional rowing exercises. It's particularly beneficial for targeting the muscles of the upper back, including the rhomboids and trapezius.

Instructions for Inverted Wall Rows

1. Starting Position: Lean back at an angle with your feet flat against the floor . Hold a resistance band that's anchored above you, keeping your arms extended.

2. Movement: Pull your upper body towards the wall by bending your elbows and squeezing your shoulder blades together. Keep your body straight and avoid sagging your hips.

3. Return: Slowly extend your arms and return to the starting position.

4. Breathing: Inhale as you extend your arms and exhale as you pull your body towards the wall.

5. Posture: Maintain a straight line from your head to your heels throughout the exercise. Engage your core for stability.

Number of Sets and Repetitions

- ☐ - Beginners: Start with 2 sets of 8 to 10 repetitions. Focus on form and control.
- ☐ - Intermediate: Perform 3 sets of 10 to 12 repetitions.
- ☐ - Advanced: Increase the challenge by adding more sets, using a heavier resistance band, or slowing down the movement.

Inverted Wall Rows are an excellent exercise for developing strength in the upper back, enhancing posture, and building overall upper body endurance. They can be easily modified to suit different fitness levels and are a great addition to any strength training routine. Remember to keep the movement controlled, focusing on engaging your back muscles throughout the exercise.

Wall Handstand Push-Ups

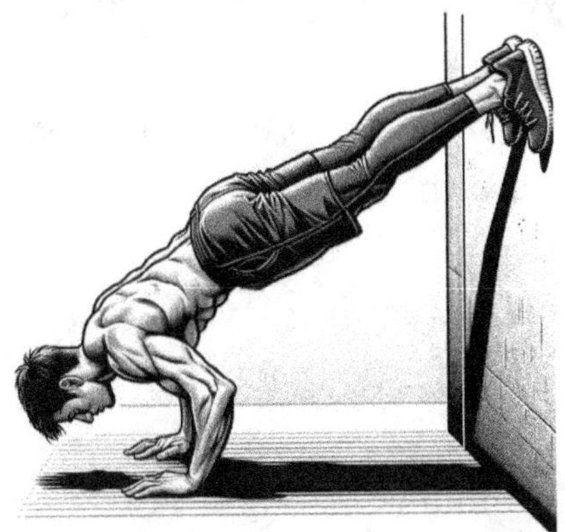

Wall Handstand Push-Ups are a challenging and advanced exercise that targets the upper body, particularly the shoulders, arms, and core. This exercise is a variation of the classic push-up, performed in a handstand position against a wall. It's ideal for those who have a strong foundation in upper body strength and are looking to take their workout to the next level.

Instructions for Wall Handstand Push-Ups

1. Starting Position: Begin in a handstand position against the wall, with your feet resting on the wall for support. Your hands should be placed on the ground, shoulder-width apart.

2. Movement: Lower your head towards the ground by bending your elbows, keeping your body straight.

3. Push Up: Push back up to the handstand position, extending your arms fully.

4. Breathing: Breathe in as you lower yourself and out as you raise yourself back up.

5. Posture: Maintain a straight body line from head to heels. Keep your core engaged to stabilize your body.

Number of Sets and Repetitions

- ☐ - Beginners: It's recommended to start with wall handstands to build strength before attempting push-ups.
- ☐ - Intermediate: Perform 2 sets of 3 to 5 repetitions, focusing on form and control.
- ☐ - Advanced: Increase to 3 sets of 6 to 8 repetitions or more, depending on your strength and experience.

Wall Handstand Push-Ups are an excellent exercise for building significant upper body strength and improving balance and coordination. They require a good level of fitness and should be attempted only after mastering basic handstands and push-ups. Remember to perform the exercise with caution and control, focusing on maintaining proper form throughout the movement.

CHAPTER 7: LOWER BODY EXERCISES

Wall Squats

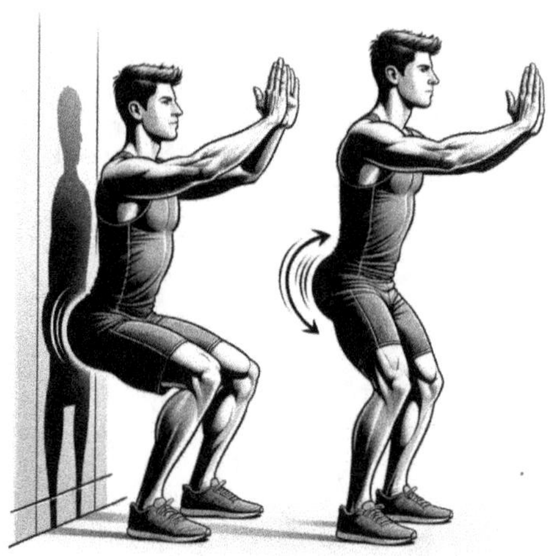

Wall Squats are a beneficial exercise for strengthening the thighs, glutes, and core muscles. This exercise provides a stable and controlled way to perform squats, making it suitable for individuals at various fitness levels, including those who may need extra support due to balance or strength limitations.

Instructions for Wall Squats

1. Starting Position: Stand with your back against a wall. Place your feet shoulder-width apart and about 2 feet away from the wall.

2. Movement: Slide down the wall into a squat position. Your knees should be bent to a 90-degree angle, and your thighs should be parallel to the floor.

3. Hold: Maintain the squat position, ensuring your back is flat against the wall. Extend your arms in front of you for balance.

4. Return: Slide back up the wall to return to the starting position.

5. Breathing: Inhale as you slide down into the squat and exhale as you slide back up.

6. Posture: Keep your weight in your heels and ensure your knees do not extend past your toes.

Number of Sets and Repetitions

- ☐ - Beginners: Start with 2 sets of 8 to 10 repetitions. Focus on form and control.
- ☐ - Intermediate: Perform 3 sets of 12 to 15 repetitions.
- ☐ - Advanced: Increase the challenge by holding the squat position for a longer duration or adding more sets.

Wall Squats are an excellent exercise for building strength in the lower body and improving posture. They are a versatile exercise that can be adapted to suit different fitness levels and goals. Remember to keep your movements controlled and focus on maintaining proper alignment throughout the exercise.

Wall Lunges

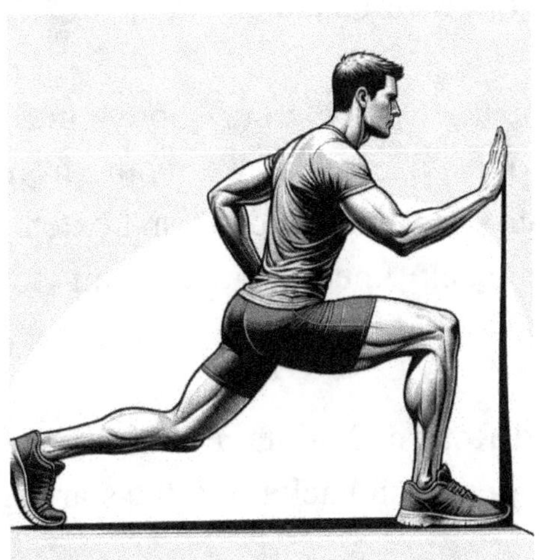

Wall Lunges are an effective lower body exercise that focuses on strengthening the quadriceps, glutes, and hamstrings. Utilizing the wall for support, this exercise variation adds stability, making it suitable for beginners or those who need extra balance assistance. It's also excellent for individuals looking to focus on form and alignment in their lunges.

Instructions for Wall Lunges

1. Starting Position: Stand with your face to the wall using your hand as support . Step one foot forward and extend the other foot back, placing the toes against the floor for balance.

2. Movement: Lower your body into a lunge, bending both knees. Ensure your front knee is aligned over your ankle and doesn't extend past your toes. Your back knee should point towards the ground.

3. Hold and Return: Maintain the lunge position for a moment, then push back up to the starting position.

4. Breathing: Inhale as you lower your body into the lunge and exhale as you push back up.

5. Posture: Keep your upper body upright and your hands on your hips for balance.

Number of Sets and Repetitions

- ☐ - Beginners: Start with 2 sets of 8 to 10 lunges on each leg. Focus on maintaining balance and proper form.

☐ - Intermediate: Perform 3 sets of 10 to 12 lunges per leg.

☐ - Advanced: Increase the challenge by holding the lunge position for a longer duration or adding more sets.

Wall Lunges are a fantastic exercise for building strength and stability in the lower body. They are particularly useful for those working on improving their lunge technique or who require additional support for balance. Remember to keep your movements controlled and focus on maintaining proper alignment throughout the exercise.

<u>Wall Sit with Calf Raises</u>

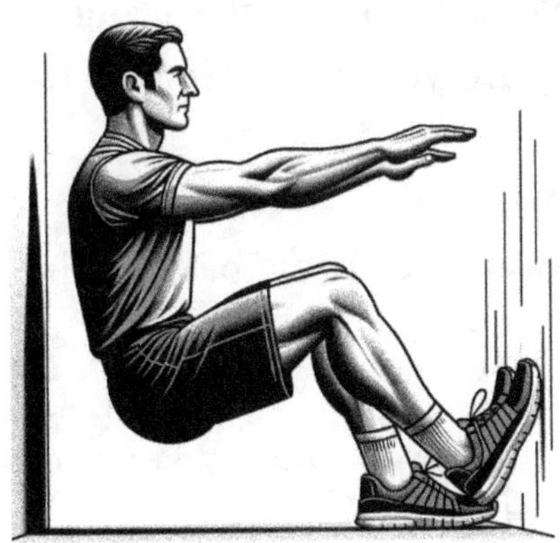

Wall Sit with Calf Raises is an effective lower body exercise that combines the benefits of wall sits with calf raises. This exercise targets the quadriceps, glutes, and calf muscles, making it a comprehensive workout for leg strength and endurance. It's particularly beneficial for enhancing stability, balance, and muscle tone in the lower body.

Instructions for Wall Sit with Calf Raises

1. Starting Position: Stand with your back flat against a wall. Slide down into a wall sit position, with your knees bent at a 90-degree angle and feet flat on the ground, shoulder-width apart.

2. Movement: While maintaining the wall sit posture, lift your heels off the ground, performing calf raises. Ensure your back remains flat against the wall.

3. Return: Lower your heels back to the ground and repeat the calf raises.

4. Breathing: Inhale as you lower your heels, and exhale as you lift them.

5. Posture: Keep your core engaged and maintain the wall sit position throughout the exercise.

Number of Sets and Repetitions

- □ - Beginners: Start with 2 sets of 10 to 12 calf raises. Focus on maintaining the wall sit posture.
- □ - Intermediate: Perform 3 sets of 15 calf raises.
- □ - Advanced: Increase the challenge by holding the calf raise position for a few seconds or adding more sets.

Wall Sit with Calf Raises is an excellent exercise for building lower body strength and endurance. This combined movement effectively works multiple muscle groups, making it a valuable addition to any fitness routine. Remember to perform the exercise with control, focusing on maintaining proper form throughout.

Wall Glute Bridges

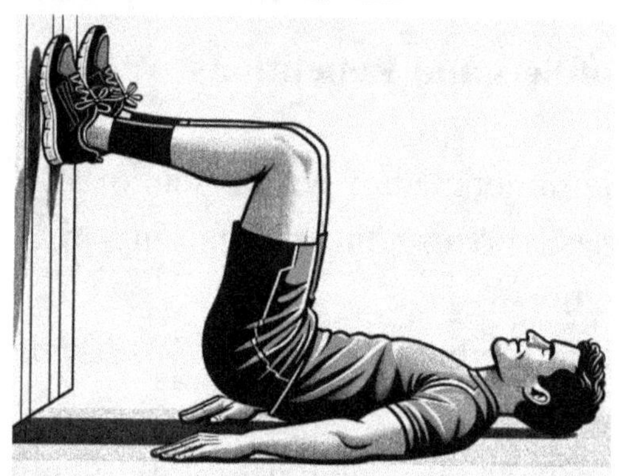

Wall Glute Bridges are an excellent exercise for targeting the glutes and hamstrings, crucial for lower body strength and stability. This exercise is beneficial for improving hip mobility, strengthening the lower back, and enhancing overall core stability. It's a great variation of the traditional glute bridge, using the wall for added resistance and support.

Instructions for Wall Glute Bridges

1. Starting Position: Lie on your back with your arms flat on the ground for support. Place your feet flat against the wall, knees bent.

2. Movement: Lift your hips off the ground, forming a straight line from your shoulders to your knees. Ensure your feet remain flat against the wall.

3. Hold and Return: Hold the raised position for a moment, then slowly lower your hips back to the starting position.

4. Breathing: Inhale as you lower your hips and exhale as you lift them upwards.

5. Posture: Keep your movements controlled and ensure your back is straight as you lift your hips.

Number of Sets and Repetitions

- ☐ - Beginners: Start with 2 sets of 8 to 10 repetitions. Focus on form and controlled movement.
- ☐ - Intermediate: Perform 3 sets of 12 to 15 repetitions.
- ☐ - Advanced: Increase the challenge by holding the raised position for a longer duration or adding more sets.

Wall Glute Bridges are an effective way to strengthen the glutes and hamstrings, improve hip mobility, and support lower back health. They are a versatile exercise that can be adapted to suit different fitness levels and goals. Remember to perform the exercise with control, focusing on engaging your glutes and maintaining proper form throughout.

Wall Supported Warrior III

Wall Supported Warrior III is a dynamic balance and strength exercise inspired by the traditional yoga pose. This variation adds the stability of a wall, making it accessible to individuals at various fitness levels. It focuses on improving balance, core strength, and lower body stability while enhancing concentration and posture.

Instructions for Wall Supported Warrior III

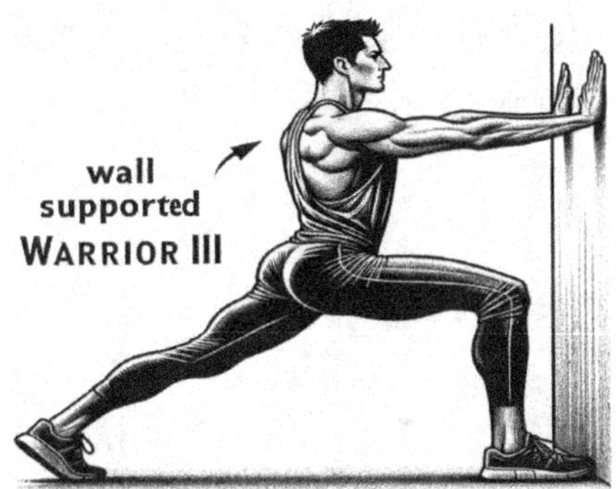

1. Starting Position: Stand facing the wall. Place your hands on the wall at shoulder height for balance.

2. Movement: Extend one leg back, lifting it off the ground. Lean forward, forming a straight line with your body and extended leg, parallel to the ground. Your supporting leg should be slightly bent.

3. Hold and Switch: Maintain the position, ensuring your body and extended leg are aligned. Hold for 10 to 20 seconds, then return to the starting position and switch legs.

4. Breathing: Inhale as you extend your leg and exhale as you hold the position. Keep your breathing steady and controlled.

5. Posture: Keep your hips square and your core engaged. Focus on maintaining a straight line from your head to your extended heel.

Number of Sets and Repetitions

- ☐ - Beginners: Start with 2 sets of 10 to 20 seconds per leg. Focus on balance and form.
- ☐ - Intermediate: Perform 3 sets, holding each pose for up to 30 seconds per leg.
- ☐ - Advanced: Increase the challenge by holding the pose for a longer duration or adding ankle weights.

Wall Supported Warrior III is a beneficial exercise for enhancing balance, core strength, and lower body stability. It's a versatile exercise that can be adapted to suit different fitness levels and goals. Remember to perform the exercise with control, focusing on maintaining proper alignment and balance throughout.

Wall Assisted Pistol Squats

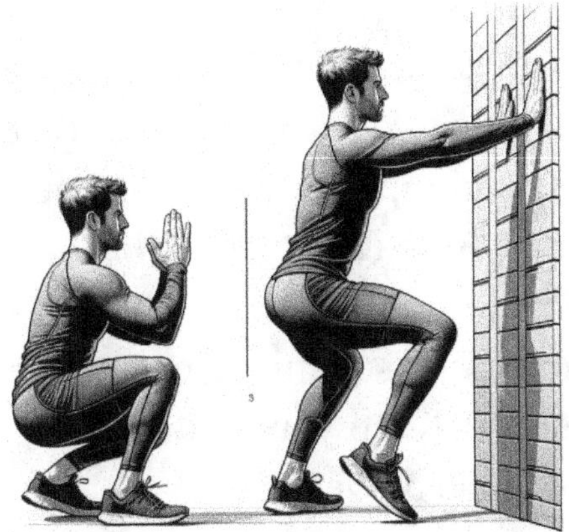

Wall Assisted Pistol Squats are a challenging lower body exercise that focuses on strength, balance, and flexibility. This exercise is a variation of the traditional pistol squat, using a wall for support. It targets the quadriceps, glutes, and hamstrings, while also testing your balance and coordination. This exercise is excellent for athletes and fitness enthusiasts looking to enhance unilateral (one-sided) strength and stability.

Instructions for Wall Assisted Pistol Squats

1. Starting Position: Stand sideways to a wall, using one hand for support. Keep your feet shoulder-width apart.

2. Movement: Lift one leg forward, keeping it straight. Perform a single-leg squat with your other leg, bending at the knee and hip to lower your body as far down as comfortably possible.

3. Return: Push through your squatting leg to rise back to the starting position. Keep your extended leg off the ground throughout the movement.

4. Breathing: Inhale as you lower into the squat and exhale as you rise back up.

5. Posture: Keep your back straight and core engaged. Use the wall for balance but try to minimize reliance on it.

Number of Sets and Repetitions

- ☐ - Beginners: Start with 2 sets of 5 to 6 repetitions per leg. Focus on balance and controlled movement.

Pg. 180

☐ - Intermediate: Perform 3 sets of 8 repetitions per leg.

☐ - Advanced: Increase the challenge by reducing hand support, adding more repetitions, or holding a weight.

Wall Assisted Pistol Squats are an effective way to build lower body strength and improve balance. They are particularly useful for athletes or individuals who require strong unilateral leg strength. Remember to perform the exercise with control, focusing on maintaining proper form and balance throughout.

Wall Hamstring Curls (Using a Stability Ball)

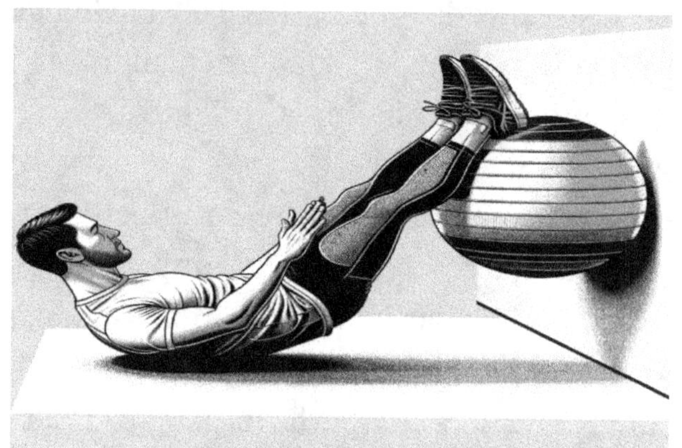

Wall Hamstring Curls with a stability ball are an effective exercise for strengthening the hamstring muscles and improving lower body stability. This exercise combines the use of a stability ball with the support of a wall, making it suitable for various fitness levels. It's excellent for targeting the hamstrings while also engaging the glutes and core muscles.

Instructions for Wall Hamstring Curls (Using a Stability Ball)

1. Starting Position: Lie on your back with your feet placed on top of a stability ball, close to the wall for

support. Keep your arms flat on the ground for balance.

2. Movement: Lift your hips off the ground, creating a straight line from your shoulders to your feet. Roll the ball towards your body by bending your knees, engaging your hamstrings.

3. Return: Slowly extend your legs, rolling the ball back to the starting position while keeping your hips lifted.

4. Breathing: Inhale as you extend your legs and exhale as you roll the ball towards your body.

5. Posture: Maintain a straight and stable spine throughout the exercise. Engage your core to support your hips and back.

Number of Sets and Repetitions

- ☐ - Beginners: Start with 2 sets of 8 to 10 repetitions. Focus on smooth movement and maintaining hip elevation.

- ☐ - Intermediate: Perform 3 sets of 10 to 12 repetitions.
- ☐ - Advanced: Increase the challenge by adding more sets or holding the curled position for a few seconds.

Wall Hamstring Curls with a stability ball are an excellent way to build strength in the hamstrings and improve overall lower body stability. This exercise can be easily adapted to different fitness levels by adjusting the number of repetitions and sets. Remember to perform the exercise with control, focusing on engaging your hamstring muscles throughout the movement.

Wall Inner Thigh Squeezes

Wall Inner Thigh Squeezes are a focused exercise for strengthening the adductor muscles of the inner thigh. This exercise is beneficial for improving hip stability and toning the inner thighs. Using a wall and a small exercise ball or pillow adds an element of resistance, making the exercise more effective.

Instructions for Wall Inner Thigh Squeezes

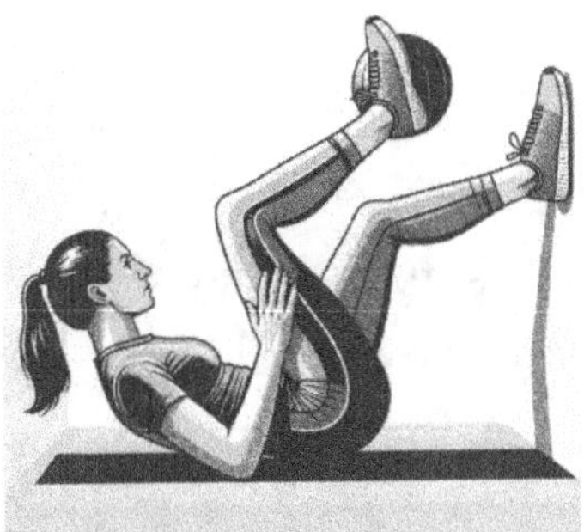

1. Starting Position: Lie on your back with your hips and legs elevated against the wall, forming a 90-degree angle with your body.

2. Movement: Place a small exercise ball or a pillow between your knees. Squeeze the ball or pillow with your knees to engage the inner thigh muscles.

3. Hold and Release: Hold the squeeze for a few seconds, then release slightly before squeezing again.

4. Breathing: Inhale as you release the squeeze and exhale as you engage your inner thigh muscles.

5. Posture: Keep your back flat on the ground and your core engaged throughout the exercise.

Number of Sets and Repetitions

- ☐ - Beginners: Start with 2 sets of 10 to 12 squeezes. Focus on controlled movements.
- ☐ - Intermediate: Perform 3 sets of 15 squeezes.
- ☐ - Advanced: Increase the challenge by holding the squeeze for a longer duration or adding more sets.

Wall Inner Thigh Squeezes are an excellent exercise for targeting the often-neglected inner thigh muscles. They are suitable for all fitness levels and can be easily incorporated into any lower body or core workout routine. Remember to perform the exercise with control, focusing on engaging your inner thigh muscles throughout the movement.

Wall Supported Hip Abductions

Wall Supported Hip Abductions are a targeted exercise for strengthening the outer thigh and hip abductor muscles. This exercise is particularly beneficial for improving hip stability and enhancing lateral leg strength. The use of a wall for support makes it accessible for various fitness levels and helps maintain proper posture during the exercise.

Instructions for Wall Supported Hip Abductions

1. Starting Position: Stand sideways to the wall, with one hand on the wall for support.

2. Movement: Lift your outer leg away from your body, keeping it straight. Focus on engaging the muscles of your outer thigh and hip.

3. Hold and Return: Hold the lifted position for a moment, then slowly lower your leg back to the starting position.

4. Breathing: Inhale as you lower your leg and exhale as you lift it.

5. Posture: Keep your body upright and avoid leaning towards the wall. Engage your core for better balance and control.

Number of Sets and Repetitions

- □ - Beginners: Start with 2 sets of 8 to 10 repetitions per leg. Focus on controlled movements.
- □ - Intermediate: Perform 3 sets of 12 repetitions per leg.
- □ - Advanced: Increase the challenge by holding the lifted position for a longer duration or adding ankle weights.

Wall Supported Hip Abductions are an effective exercise for targeting the hip abductor muscles, essential for lateral movements and overall hip stability. They can be incorporated into lower body workout routines or used as a standalone exercise for hip strengthening. Remember to perform the exercise with control, focusing on engaging the correct muscles and maintaining proper posture throughout.

Wall Supported Hip Abductions

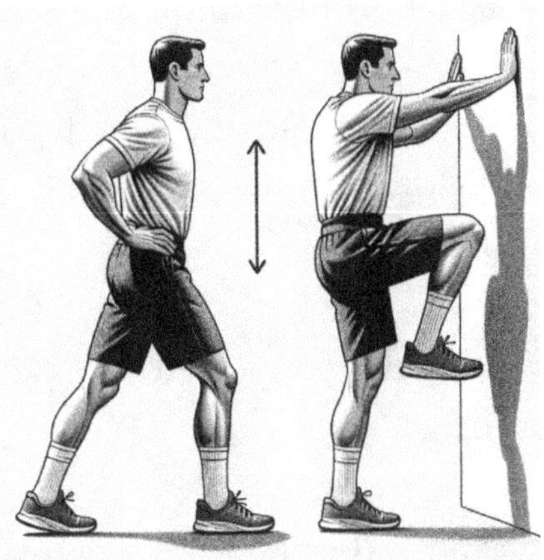

Wall Supported Hip Abductions are a targeted exercise for strengthening the outer thigh and hip abductor muscles. This exercise is particularly beneficial for improving hip stability and enhancing lateral leg strength. The use of a wall for support makes it accessible for various fitness levels and helps maintain proper posture during the exercise.

Instructions for Wall Supported Hip Abductions

1. Starting Position: Stand sideways to the wall, with one hand on the wall for support.

2. Movement: Lift your outer leg away from your body, keeping it straight. Focus on engaging the muscles of your outer thigh and hip.

3. Hold and Return: Hold the lifted position for a moment, then slowly lower your leg back to the starting position.

4. Breathing: Inhale as you lower your leg and exhale as you lift it.

5. Posture: Keep your body upright and avoid leaning towards the wall. Engage your core for better balance and control.

Number of Sets and Repetitions

- ☐ - Beginners: Start with 2 sets of 8 to 10 repetitions per leg. Focus on controlled movements.
- ☐ - Intermediate: Perform 3 sets of 12 repetitions per leg.
- ☐ - Advanced: Increase the challenge by holding the lifted position for a longer duration or adding ankle weights.

Wall Supported Hip Abductions are an effective exercise for targeting the hip abductor muscles, essential for lateral movements and overall hip stability. They can be incorporated into lower body workout routines or used as a standalone exercise for hip strengthening. Remember to perform the exercise with control, focusing on engaging the correct muscles and maintaining proper posture throughout.

<u>Wall Slide Leg Lifts</u>

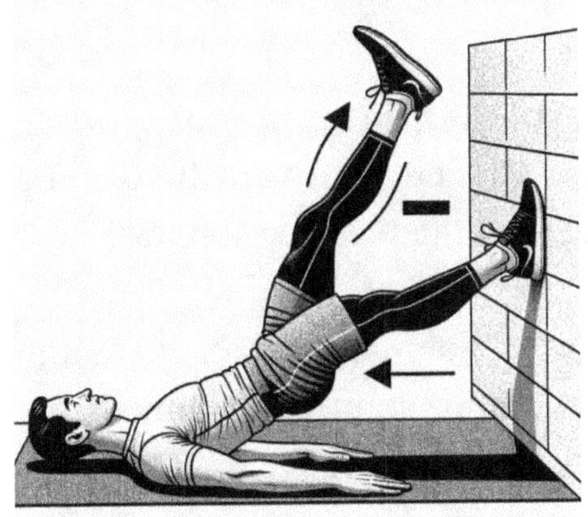

Wall Slide Leg Lifts are an effective lower body exercise designed to strengthen the hip abductor muscles and improve leg flexibility. This exercise is particularly beneficial for those seeking to enhance their side leg strength and stability. Performing this exercise against a wall ensures proper form and alignment, making it suitable for all fitness levels.

Instructions for Wall Slide Leg Lifts

1. Starting Position: Lie on your side with your back and legs straight against the wall. Your body should form a straight line.

2. Movement: Lift your top leg upwards while keeping it straight and aligned with your body. The bottom leg remains against the wall for support.

3. Return: Slowly lower your top leg back to the starting position, maintaining control throughout the movement.

4. Breathing: Inhale as you lower your leg and exhale as you lift it.

5. Posture: Keep your core engaged and your body straight to ensure proper alignment.

Number of Sets and Repetitions

- ☐ - Beginners: Start with 2 sets of 8 to 10 repetitions per leg. Focus on maintaining alignment and control.
- ☐ - Intermediate: Perform 3 sets of 12 to 15 repetitions per leg.
- ☐ - Advanced: Increase the challenge by holding the lifted position for a few seconds or adding ankle weights.

Wall Slide Leg Lifts are an excellent way to target the muscles in the outer thigh and hip area. They can be easily incorporated into lower body workout routines or used as a standalone exercise for leg strengthening. Remember to perform the exercise with control, focusing on engaging the correct muscles and maintaining proper posture throughout.

CHAPTER 8: POSTURE AND BALANCE EXERCISES

Wall Plank

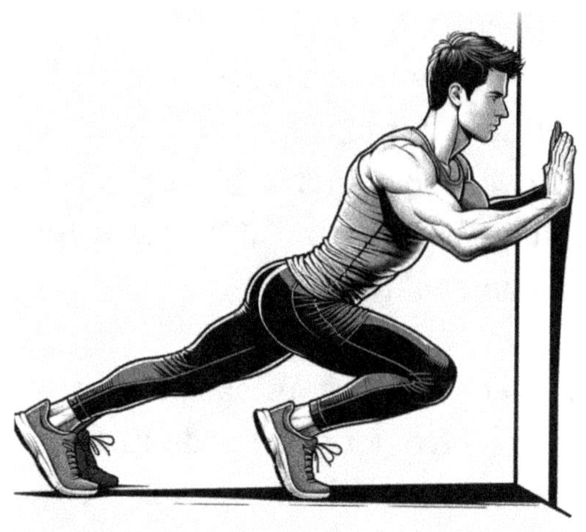

The Wall Plank is a variation of the traditional floor plank, offering a different level of intensity while targeting core stability and strength. This exercise is excellent for engaging the entire core, shoulders, and back, promoting good posture and overall muscle endurance.

Instructions for Wall Plank

1. Starting Position: Face the wall and place your forearms on the wall at shoulder height. Step back from the wall until your body is in a straight line from your head to your heels.

2. Movement: Engage your core, glutes, and shoulders to maintain a stable plank position. Keep your body straight, and avoid sagging your hips or raising your buttocks.

3. Hold: Maintain the plank position for the desired duration, focusing on keeping your core engaged and your body aligned.

4. Breathing: Breathe steadily and deeply throughout the exercise. Focus on maintaining a tight core and controlled breathing.

5. Posture: Ensure your elbows are directly under your shoulders and your head is in a neutral position.

Number of Sets and Repetitions

Pg. 195

- ☐ - Beginners: Start with holding the plank for 20 to 30 seconds. Perform 2 sets.
- ☐ - Intermediate: Hold the plank for 45 to 60 seconds. Perform 2 to 3 sets.
- ☐ - Advanced: Increase the duration of the hold or add additional sets for a greater challenge.

The Wall Plank is a versatile and effective exercise for building core strength and improving overall stability. It's suitable for individuals of all fitness levels and can be easily modified by adjusting the duration of the hold. Remember to perform the exercise with control, focusing on maintaining proper form and alignment throughout.

Wall Pelvic Tilts

Wall Pelvic Tilts are a gentle yet effective exercise designed to engage and strengthen the core and lower back muscles. This exercise promotes pelvic mobility, helps alleviate lower back tension, and can contribute to improved posture. It's especially beneficial for individuals looking to enhance core stability and for those who may experience lower back discomfort.

Instructions for Wall Pelvic Tilts

1. Starting Position: Stand with your back against the wall, feet shoulder-width apart and slightly away from the wall. Your arms should be relaxed by your sides or placed on your hips or lower back for support.

2. Movement: Gently tilt your pelvis forward, tightening your abdominal muscles and flattening your lower back against the wall. Then, tilt your pelvis backward, arching your lower back slightly away from the wall.

3. Hold and Release: Hold each tilt for a few seconds, then release and return to the neutral starting position.

4. Breathing: Inhale as you tilt your pelvis backward and exhale as you tilt it forward.

5. Posture: Keep your upper body still and focused on the movement of your pelvis. Your spine should remain in a neutral position throughout the exercise.

Number of Sets and Repetitions

- ☐ - Beginners: Start with 2 sets of 10 to 12 tilts. Focus on controlled movement and engaging your core.
- ☐ - Intermediate: Perform 3 sets of 15 tilts.
- ☐ - Advanced: Increase the challenge by holding the tilt position for a longer duration or adding more sets.

Wall Pelvic Tilts are an excellent exercise for improving pelvic mobility, strengthening the core, and alleviating lower back tension. They are suitable for all fitness levels and can be easily incorporated into any workout routine or performed as a standalone exercise. Remember to perform the exercise with control, focusing on engaging your pelvic and core muscles throughout the movement.

Standing Wall Calf Raises

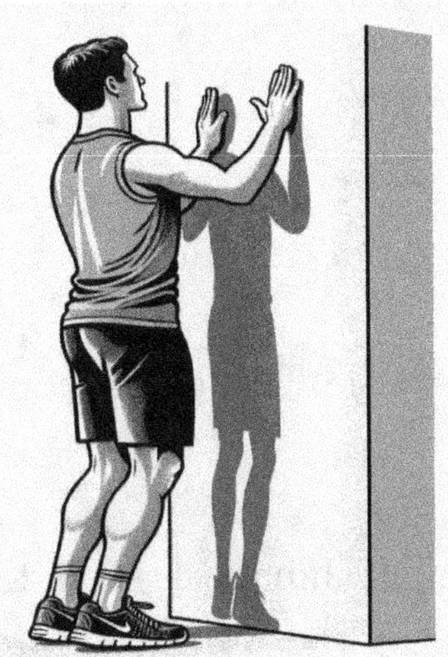

Standing Wall Calf Raises are a simple and effective exercise for strengthening the calf muscles. This exercise is excellent for enhancing lower leg strength, improving balance, and can contribute to better stability and support for various physical activities. It's a versatile workout that can be done anywhere with wall support, making it suitable for all fitness levels.

Instructions for Standing Wall Calf Raises

1. Starting Position: Stand facing a wall with your hands resting on the wall for balance. Keep your feet flat on the ground, about hip-width apart.

2. Movement: Rise onto the toes of your feet, lifting your heels off the ground. Focus on engaging and tightening your calf muscles.

3. Return: Slowly lower your heels back to the ground.

4. Breathing: Inhale as you lower your heels and exhale as you rise onto your toes.

5. Posture: Keep your body straight and avoid bending at the hips or knees. Use the wall for balance but not for support.

Number of Sets and Repetitions

- ☐ - Beginners: Start with 2 sets of 10 to 12 raises. Focus on controlled movements.
- ☐ - Intermediate: Perform 3 sets of 15 to 20 raises.

☐ - Advanced: Increase the challenge by holding at the top position for a few seconds or adding more sets.

Standing Wall Calf Raises are an excellent way to target the muscles in your calves, essential for walking, running, and maintaining balance. They can be easily incorporated into any fitness routine or performed as a standalone exercise for lower leg strengthening. Remember to perform the exercise with control, focusing on engaging your calf muscles throughout the movement.

Wall Tree Pose

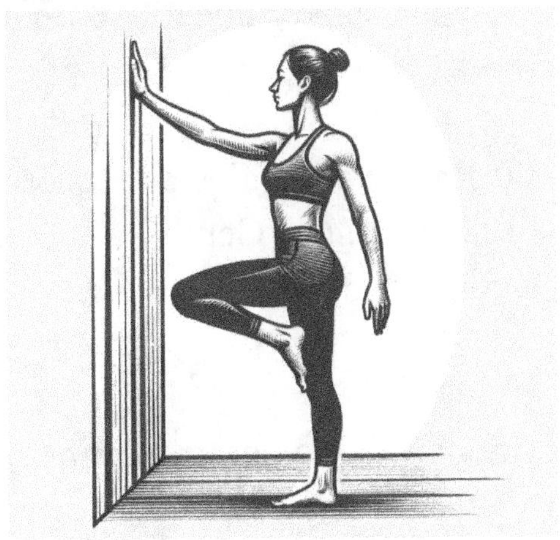

The Wall Tree Pose is a modified version of the classic Tree Pose (Vrksasana) in yoga, adapted for additional stability and support using a wall. This pose is excellent for enhancing balance, focusing the mind, and strengthening the ankles, legs, and core. It's particularly beneficial for beginners or those who need extra support in balancing poses.

Instructions for Wall Tree Pose

1. Starting Position: Stand facing the wall with one hand resting on the wall for balance.

2. Movement: Shift your weight onto the leg closest to the wall. Place the sole of your other foot on the inner thigh of your standing leg, avoiding the knee joint.

3. Alignment: Ensure your hips are square and your standing leg is straight. Gently press your foot against your thigh and your thigh against your foot for stability.

4. Arm Position: Raise your free arm upwards or place it on your hip. If you feel stable, you can try bringing both arms up over your head.

Pg. 202

5. Hold and Switch: Maintain the pose for 30 seconds to 1 minute, focusing on your breath and balance. Gently release and switch sides.

6. Breathing: Breathe deeply and steadily throughout the pose, focusing on maintaining a calm and centered state.

Number of Sets and Repetitions

- ☐ - Frequency: This pose can be practiced daily as part of a yoga or balance routine.
- ☐ - Duration: Hold the pose for 30 seconds to 1 minute on each side, depending on your comfort and balance.

The Wall Tree Pose is a versatile and accessible exercise that improves balance, concentration, and overall body alignment. It's a great way to build confidence in balancing poses and can be a calming addition to any fitness or yoga practice. Remember to perform the pose with control, focusing on maintaining proper alignment and steady breathing throughout.

Wall Warrior Pose

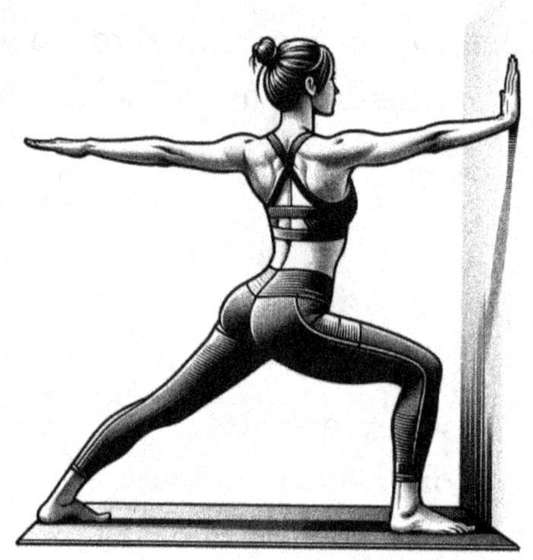

The Wall Warrior Pose is a variation of the traditional yoga Warrior Pose (Virabhadrasana). This adaptation provides extra support and stability, making it ideal for improving balance, leg strength, and flexibility. The wall support helps in maintaining correct posture, which is beneficial for beginners or those working on their alignment.

Instructions for Wall Warrior Pose

1. Starting Position: Stand facing the wall. Step one foot forward and extend the other foot back, placing the heel down.

2. Movement: Bend your front kneel, ensuring it is aligned over your ankle. Keep your back leg straight with the heel slightly lifted up

3. Arm Position: Extend your arms at shoulder height, parallel to the ground with one touching the wall.

4. Hold and Switch: Maintain the pose for the recommended duration. Release and switch your leg position to repeat on the other side.

5. Breathing: Breathe deeply and steadily, focusing on maintaining a strong and stable stance.

Number of Sets and Repetitions

- ☐ - Beginners: Hold the pose for 20 to 30 seconds on each side. Perform 1 to 2 sets.
- ☐ - Intermediate: Hold for 45 to 60 seconds on each side. Perform 2 to 3 sets.

☐ - Advanced: Increase the duration of the hold or add additional sets for a greater challenge.

The Wall Warrior Pose is effective for enhancing leg strength, improving balance, and opening the hips and chest. Performing this pose with the back against the wall helps in building confidence in standing poses and ensures proper alignment. Remember to perform the pose with control, focusing on maintaining proper alignment and steady breathing throughout.

Wall-Assisted Single Leg Deadlift

The Wall-Assisted Single Leg Deadlift is a functional exercise that focuses on improving balance, coordination, and strength in the lower body, particularly targeting the hamstrings and glutes. This exercise variation incorporates wall support to enhance stability, making it suitable for various fitness levels, including beginners or those recovering from injury.

Instructions for Wall-Assisted Single Leg Deadlift

1. Starting Position: Stand on one leg, with the other leg extended straight back and your hand on the wall for balance.

2. Movement: Bend forward at the waist while keeping your standing leg slightly bent. Reach your free hand towards the ground, creating a T-shape with your body. Keep your back straight and your extended leg in line with your body.

3. Return: Slowly return to the starting position, maintaining balance and control throughout the movement.

4. Breathing: Inhale as you bend forward and exhale as you return to the starting position.

5. Posture: Keep your hips square and your core engaged to maintain stability.

Number of Sets and Repetitions

☐ - Beginners: Start with 2 sets of 6 to 8 repetitions per leg. Focus on form and maintaining balance.

☐ - Intermediate: Perform 3 sets of 8 to 10 repetitions per leg.

☐ - Advanced: Increase the challenge by holding the bent position for a few seconds or adding more sets.

The Wall-Assisted Single Leg Deadlift is an excellent exercise for developing balance, hamstring flexibility, and glute strength. It's beneficial for enhancing overall lower body stability and can be adapted to suit different fitness levels and goals. Remember to perform the exercise with control, focusing on maintaining proper form and balance throughout.

Wall Supported Triangle Pose

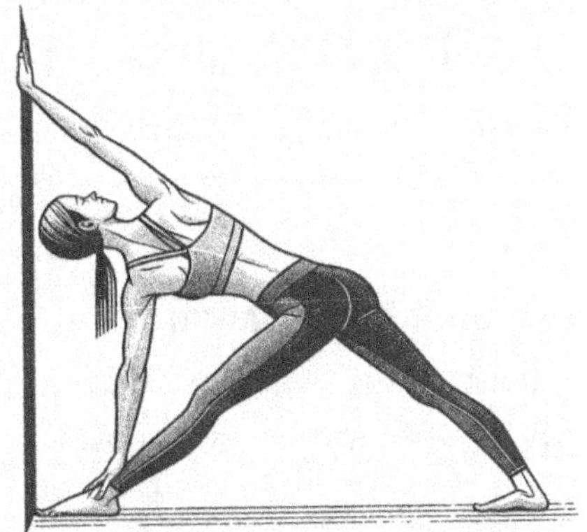

The Wall Supported Triangle Pose is a variation of the classic Triangle Pose (Trikonasana) in yoga, modified to provide stability and alignment using a wall. This pose is excellent for stretching the sides of the waist, strengthening the legs, and improving overall balance and concentration. The wall support makes this pose accessible to beginners or those working on their balance and flexibility.

Instructions for Wall Supported Triangle Pose

1. Starting Position: Stand facing the wall, legs wide apart. Extend your arms at shoulder height, parallel to the ground.

2. Movement: Turn one foot out 90 degrees and the other foot in slightly. Reach the hand of your turned-out foot down towards your ankle, and extend the other hand up towards the ceiling or the wall if comfortable.

3. Alignment: Ensure your torso is straight and aligned with your legs, forming a triangle shape with your body. The wall will help maintain this alignment.

4. Hold and Switch: Hold the pose for 30 seconds to 1 minute. Gently come up and switch sides.

5. Breathing: Breathe deeply and steadily throughout the pose, focusing on expanding your ribs with each breath.

Number of Sets and Repetitions

- ☐ - Frequency: This pose can be practiced daily as part of a yoga or flexibility routine.
- ☐ - Duration: Hold the pose for 30 seconds to 1 minute on each side, depending on your comfort and balance.

Wall Supported Triangle Pose is a beneficial exercise for enhancing flexibility, improving balance, and strengthening the legs. It's a great way to build confidence in standing poses and ensures proper alignment. Remember to perform the pose with control, focusing on maintaining proper alignment and steady breathing throughout.

Wall Supported Chair Pose

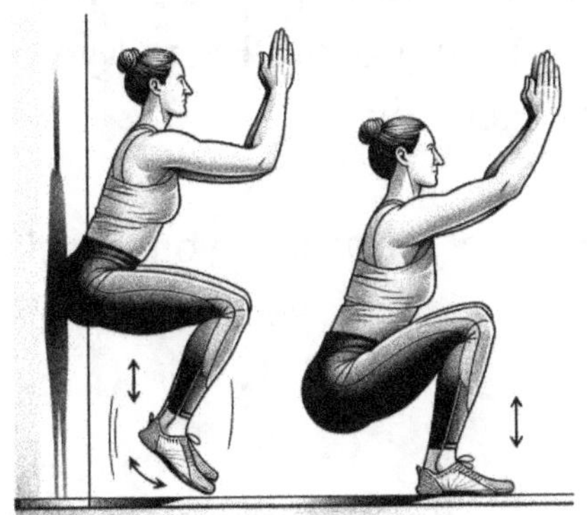

The Wall Supported Chair Pose is a variation of the traditional Chair Pose (Utkatasana) in yoga, performed with the support of a wall. This exercise is great for strengthening the thighs, glutes, and core, while also improving posture and balance. The wall provides stability and helps maintain proper form, making it accessible for beginners or those focusing on alignment.

Instructions for Wall Supported Chair Pose

1. Starting Position: Stand with your back against the wall, feet hip-width apart and a few inches away from the wall.

2. Movement: Slide down the wall into a squat position, as if sitting in an invisible chair. Your thighs should be parallel to the ground. Extend your arms upwards, parallel to each other.

3. Hold: Maintain the pose, ensuring your back remains flat against the wall. Keep your weight in your heels.

4. Breathing: Breathe deeply and steadily throughout the pose, focusing on maintaining a strong and stable squat position.

5. Posture: Keep your core engaged and your spine long. Avoid arching your lower back.

Number of Sets and Repetitions

- ☐ - Beginners: Hold the pose for 20 to 30 seconds. Perform 2 sets.
- ☐ - Intermediate: Increase the duration to 45 to 60 seconds. Perform 2 to 3 sets.
- ☐ - Advanced: Add more sets or increase the duration of the hold for a greater challenge.

Wall Supported Chair Pose is an excellent exercise for building strength in the lower body and enhancing core stability. It's suitable for individuals of all fitness levels and can be easily incorporated into a yoga or fitness routine. Remember to perform the pose with control, focusing on maintaining proper alignment and steady breathing throughout.

Wall Heel-to-Toe Stand

The Wall Heel-to-Toe Stand is a balance and coordination exercise that mimics the action of walking on a tightrope. This exercise is excellent for improving balance, coordination, and concentration. It's particularly beneficial for older adults, athletes, or anyone looking to enhance their stability and proprioceptive skills.

Instructions for Wall Heel-to-Toe Stand

1. Starting Position: Stand sideways next to a wall with one hand lightly touching the wall for balance.

2. Movement: Place one foot directly in front of the other, heel to toe, as if you are walking on a tightrope. Try to maintain this position with minimal support from the wall.

3. Arm Position: Extend your arms to the sides for added balance or use the wall for support as needed.

4. Hold and Switch: Hold the position for 20 to 30 seconds, focusing on maintaining balance. Switch your feet and repeat.

5. Breathing: Breathe normally, focusing on staying relaxed and centered.

6. Posture: Keep your body upright and your gaze forward to help maintain balance.

Number of Sets and Repetitions

- ☐ - Beginners: Hold each position for 20 to 30 seconds. Perform 2 sets on each side.
- ☐ - Intermediate: Increase the duration to 45 to 60 seconds. Perform 2 to 3 sets on each side.
- ☐ - Advanced: Challenge yourself by closing your eyes or adding more sets.

The Wall Heel-to-Toe Stand is a simple yet effective exercise for enhancing balance and coordination. It can be incorporated into a daily routine to improve stability and is particularly useful for fall prevention in older adults. Remember to perform the exercise with control, focusing on maintaining your balance throughout.

CHAPTER 9: MOBILITY EXERCISES

Wall-Assisted Squat to Toe Touch

Wall-Assisted Squat to Toe Touch is a dynamic exercise that combines the benefits of a traditional squat with the flexibility of a toe touch. This exercise is designed to strengthen the lower body, enhance flexibility in the hamstrings, and engage the core. It's particularly beneficial for improving overall balance and coordination.

Instructions for Wall-Assisted Squat to Toe Touch

1. Starting Position: Stand with your back against the wall, feet shoulder-width apart.

2. Squat Movement: Perform a squat by bending your knees and sliding down the wall. Keep your

weight in your heels and your back flat against the wall.

3. Rising and Toe Touch: As you rise from the squat, lift one leg straight in front of you. Reach with the opposite hand towards the toe of the lifted leg, engaging your core and stretching your hamstrings.

4. Return: Lower your leg back down and slide into the next squat.

5. Breathing: Inhale as you squat down and exhale as you rise and reach towards your toe.

6. Posture: Keep your core engaged and your back straight throughout the exercise. Ensure your squats are controlled and your toe touches are deliberate.

Number of Sets and Repetitions

- □ - Beginners: Start with 2 sets of 8 to 10 repetitions. Focus on form and controlled movements.
- □ - Intermediate: Perform 3 sets of 10 to 12 repetitions.

☐ - Advanced: Increase the challenge by adding more sets or holding the toe touch position for a few seconds.

The Wall-Assisted Squat to Toe Touch is an excellent exercise for building strength, improving flexibility, and enhancing balance. It's a versatile workout that targets multiple muscle groups and can be adapted to suit different fitness levels. Remember to perform the exercise with control, focusing on maintaining proper form and alignment throughout.

Wall Angel Wings

Wall Angel Wings are a gentle yet effective exercise designed to improve shoulder mobility and strengthen the upper back muscles. This exercise, often referred to as "wall angels," is excellent for correcting posture, relieving tension in the shoulder area, and enhancing overall upper body flexibility.

Instructions for Wall Angel Wings

1. Starting Position: Stand with your back against the wall, feet slightly away from the wall. Raise your arms to the sides at shoulder height with your elbows bent, as if forming the letter 'W'.

2. Movement: Slide your arms up against the wall, extending them overhead, mimicking the motion of angel wings. Keep your back, elbows, and hands in contact with the wall throughout the movement.

3. Return: Slowly slide your arms back down to the starting position.

4. Breathing: Inhale as you slide your arms up and exhale as you return them to the starting position.

5. Posture: Ensure your back remains flat against the wall. Engage your core to maintain a neutral spine.

Number of Sets and Repetitions

- ☐ - Beginners: Start with 2 sets of 8 to 10 repetitions. Focus on controlled movements and maintaining contact with the wall.
- ☐ - Intermediate: Perform 3 sets of 10 to 12 repetitions.
- ☐ - Advanced: Increase the challenge by adding more sets or holding the top position for a few seconds.

Wall Angel Wings are an excellent exercise for anyone looking to improve their posture, enhance shoulder mobility, and strengthen the upper back muscles. They are suitable for all fitness levels and can be easily incorporated into any workout routine focused on upper body flexibility and strength. Remember to perform the exercise with control, focusing on maintaining proper form and alignment throughout.

Wall-Assisted Lateral Lunges

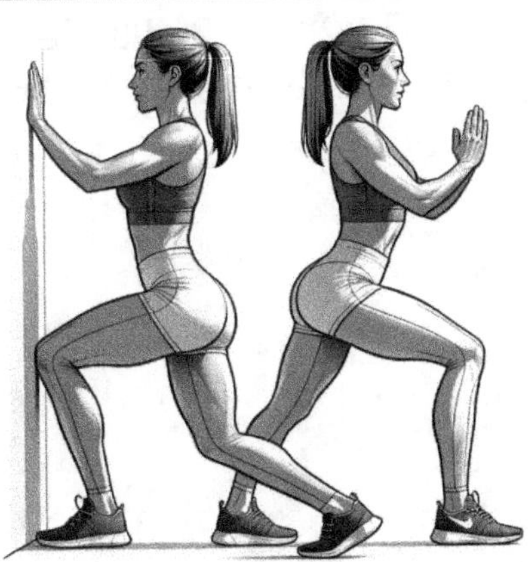

Wall-Assisted Lateral Lunges are an excellent exercise for improving flexibility and strength in the hips, glutes, and inner thigh muscles. This variation, with the support of a wall, helps maintain balance and ensures proper form, making it suitable for beginners or those looking to focus on technique.

Instructions for Wall-Assisted Lateral Lunges

1. Starting Position: Stand sideways next to a wall or stand facing the wall any position will do. Use one hand for support on the wall.

2. Movement: Step out to the side into a lunge, bending the knee of your stepping leg while keeping the other leg straight. Ensure your bent knee does not extend past your toes.

3. Return: Push off your bent leg to return to the starting position. Keep your torso upright throughout the movement.

4. Breathing: Inhale as you step into the lunge and exhale as you return to the starting position.

5. Posture: Keep your back straight and your gaze forward. Use the wall for balance, but try to minimize reliance on it.

Number of Sets and Repetitions

- □ - Beginners: Start with 2 sets of 8 to 10 lunges on each side. Focus on form and controlled movement.

Pg. 222

☐ - Intermediate: Perform 3 sets of 10 to 12 lunges per side.

☐ - Advanced: Increase the challenge by adding more sets or holding the lunge position for a few seconds.

Wall-Assisted Lateral Lunges are a versatile exercise for targeting the muscles of the inner thighs and hips. They can be easily incorporated into lower body workout routines or used as a standalone exercise for leg strengthening and flexibility. Remember to perform the exercise with control, focusing on maintaining proper form and alignment throughout.

Standing Wall Figure Eights with Arms

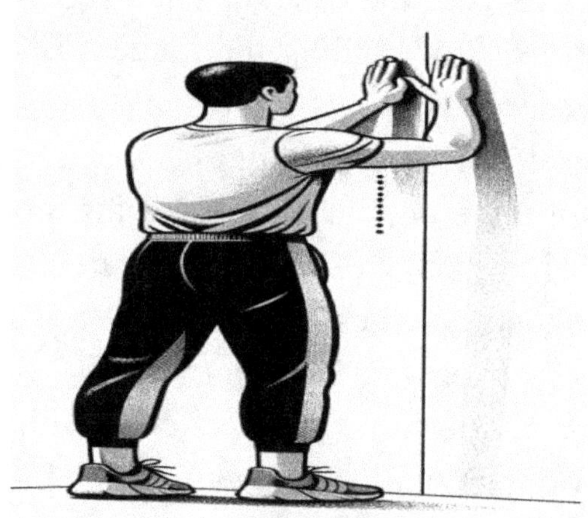

Standing Wall Figure Eights with Arms is an upper body exercise that focuses on improving shoulder mobility and enhancing coordination. This exercise involves creating figure-eight patterns with your arms against a wall, which helps to engage and strengthen the shoulder and upper back muscles. It's also beneficial for developing spatial awareness and fluid arm movements.

Instructions for Standing Wall Figure Eights with Arms

1. Starting Position: Stand facing a wall with your feet shoulder-width apart. Extend your arms and place your hands on the wall.

2. Movement: Move your arms in a fluid figure-eight pattern on the wall. Keep your movements controlled and focus on using your shoulder muscles.

3. Body Alignment: Lean your body slightly forward for balance, ensuring your feet are planted firmly on the ground.

4. Breathing: Breathe naturally, coordinating your breath with the movement of your arms.

5. Posture: Keep your back straight and your core engaged throughout the exercise.

Number of Sets and Repetitions

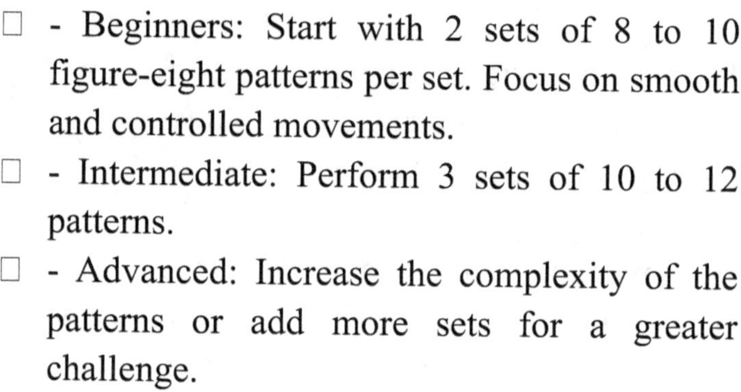

- ☐ - Beginners: Start with 2 sets of 8 to 10 figure-eight patterns per set. Focus on smooth and controlled movements.
- ☐ - Intermediate: Perform 3 sets of 10 to 12 patterns.
- ☐ - Advanced: Increase the complexity of the patterns or add more sets for a greater challenge.

Standing Wall Figure Eights with Arms is an excellent exercise for improving upper body mobility and coordination. It can be incorporated into warm-up routines or used as a standalone exercise for shoulder health. Remember to perform the exercise with control, focusing on engaging your upper body muscles throughout the movement.

Wall Supported Hip Circles with Arms

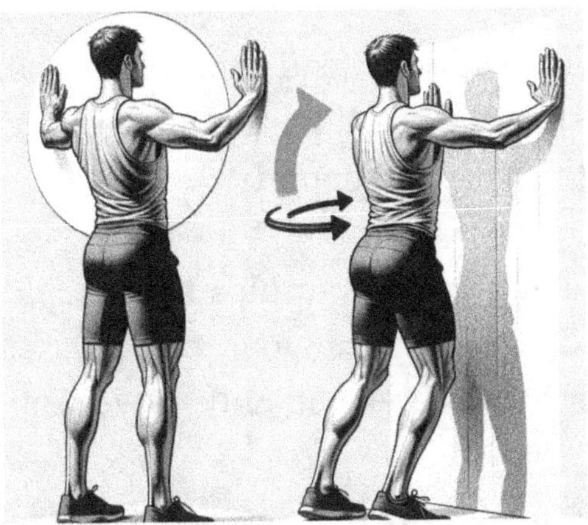

Wall Supported Hip Circles with Arms is a dynamic exercise designed to improve hip mobility and core stability. This exercise involves performing circular movements with the hips while using the wall for support, which helps maintain upper body stability. It's beneficial for those looking to enhance hip flexibility, core strength, and coordination.

Instructions for Wall Supported Hip Circles with Arms

1. Starting Position: Stand facing the wall. Extend your arms out at shoulder height with your palms touching the wall for support.

2. Movement: Rotate your hips in a circular motion, making sure to engage your core muscles. Keep your upper body stable and only move your hips.

3. Direction: Perform hip circles in both clockwise and counterclockwise directions for balanced muscle engagement.

4. Breathing: Coordinate your breathing with the movement, inhaling and exhaling smoothly throughout the exercise.

5. Posture: Keep your arms steady and your back straight. Focus on smooth, controlled hip rotations.

Number of Sets and Repetitions

- ☐ - Beginners: Start with 2 sets of 8 to 10 circles in each direction.
- ☐ - Intermediate: Perform 3 sets of 10 to 12 circles per direction.
- ☐ - Advanced: Increase the number of sets or the complexity of the hip movements for a greater challenge.

Wall Supported Hip Circles with Arms is an excellent exercise for anyone seeking to improve hip mobility and core stability. It's suitable for various fitness levels and can be easily incorporated into a warm-up routine or as part of a core and flexibility workout. Remember to perform the exercise with control, focusing on engaging your hip and core muscles throughout the movement.

Wall-Assisted Bird Dog with Arms

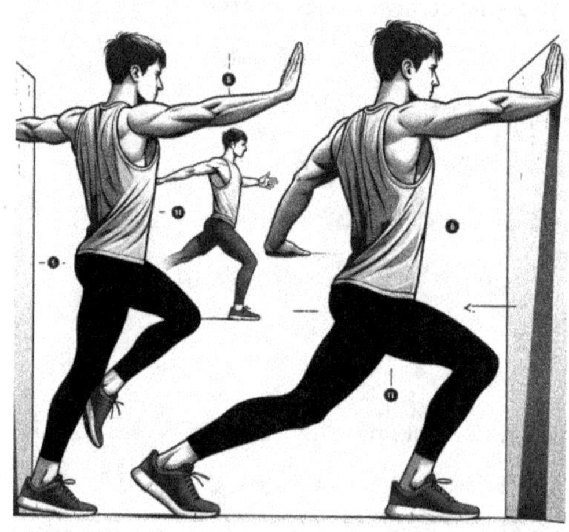

The Wall-Assisted Bird Dog with Arms is a modified version of the classic Bird Dog exercise, designed to improve core stability, balance, and coordination. Using the wall for support allows individuals to focus on the proper form and muscle engagement, making it suitable for beginners or those recovering from injury.

Instructions for Wall-Assisted Bird Dog with Arms

1. Starting Position: Stand facing the wall, placing your hands on the wall at shoulder height.

2. Movement: Extend one arm forward and the opposite leg backward, maintaining balance and engaging your core muscles. Keep your extended arm and leg in line with your body.

3. Hold and Switch: Hold the extended position for a few seconds, then return to the starting position and repeat with the opposite arm and leg.

4. Breathing: Inhale as you extend your arm and leg, and exhale as you return to the starting position.

5. Posture: Keep your back straight and your gaze forward. Ensure your movements are controlled and focused.

Number of Sets and Repetitions

- ☐ - Beginners: Start with 2 sets of 6 to 8 repetitions on each side. Focus on maintaining balance and engaging your core.
- ☐ - Intermediate: Perform 3 sets of 8 to 10 repetitions per side.
- ☐ - Advanced: Increase the hold duration for each extension or add more sets for a greater challenge.

The Wall-Assisted Bird Dog with Arms is an excellent exercise for building core strength, improving balance, and enhancing body coordination. It's adaptable for various fitness levels and can be easily incorporated into a core workout or a full-body routine. Remember to perform the exercise with control, focusing on maintaining proper form and alignment throughout.

Wall-Assisted T-spine Rotation

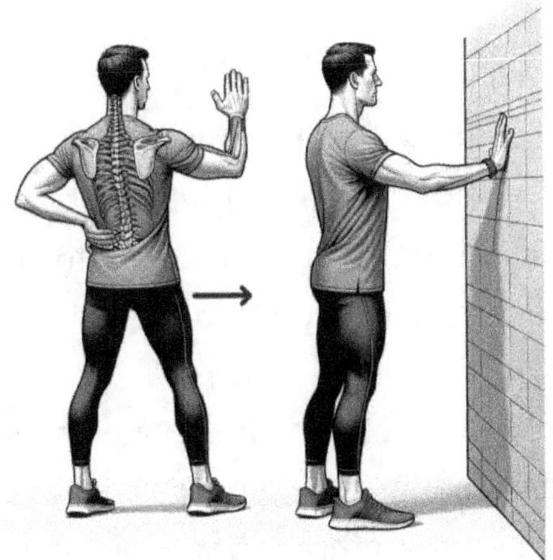

Wall-Assisted T-spine Rotation is a beneficial exercise for increasing mobility in the thoracic spine (upper back) and improving overall posture. This exercise targets the muscles responsible for rotational movements of the upper body, making it ideal for those looking to enhance their spinal flexibility and alleviate stiffness in the upper back.

Instructions for Wall-Assisted T-spine Rotation

1. Starting Position: Stand sideways next to the wall with your closer hand resting on the wall for support.

2. Movement: Rotate your upper body towards the wall while keeping your hips square and stable. Extend your other arm outwards to deepen the stretch and enhance the rotation.

3. Hold and Return: Hold the rotated position for a few seconds, feeling the stretch in your thoracic spine. Then, slowly return to the starting position.

4. Breathing: Inhale as you prepare to rotate and exhale as you perform the rotation.

5. Posture: Keep your hips stable and avoid rotating them. Focus on isolating the movement in your upper back.

Number of Sets and Repetitions

- ☐ - Beginners: Start with 2 sets of 6 to 8 rotations on each side. Focus on controlled movements and feeling the stretch in your upper back.
- ☐ - Intermediate: Perform 3 sets of 8 to 10 rotations per side.
- ☐ - Advanced: Increase the duration of the hold for each rotation or add more sets for a greater challenge.

Wall-Assisted T-spine Rotation is an excellent exercise for improving thoracic mobility, relieving tension in the upper back, and enhancing overall spinal health. It's suitable for various fitness levels and can be easily incorporated into any workout routine focused on flexibility and mobility. Remember to perform the exercise with control, focusing on maintaining proper form and alignment throughout.

Wall Balance on One Leg

Wall Balance on One Leg is a stability exercise aimed at improving balance, coordination, and core strength. This exercise is excellent for those looking to enhance their proprioceptive abilities, which is the body's ability to sense movement and position. It's particularly beneficial for athletes, older adults, or anyone seeking to improve their overall stability.

Instructions for Wall Balance on One Leg

1. Starting Position: Stand sideways next to the wall with your hand gently resting on the wall for support.

2. Movement: Shift your weight onto one leg, lifting the other leg off the ground. Hold the lifted leg in a comfortable position, ensuring your hip and knee are aligned.

3. Hold and Focus: Maintain an upright posture, keeping your core engaged. Focus your gaze forward to help maintain balance.

4. Breathing: Breathe steadily and deeply, concentrating on maintaining a stable and balanced position.

5. Posture: Keep your standing leg slightly bent to avoid locking your knee. Ensure your body is aligned and your core is activated.

Number of Sets and Repetitions

- ☐ - Beginners: Hold the balance for 20 to 30 seconds on each leg. Perform 2 sets.
- ☐ - Intermediate: Increase the duration to 45 to 60 seconds. Perform 2 to 3 sets.
- ☐ - Advanced: Challenge yourself by closing your eyes or adding arm movements.

Wall Balance on One Leg is an effective exercise for developing balance, strengthening the core, and enhancing focus. It's suitable for individuals of all fitness levels and can be easily incorporated into any workout routine focused on stability and core strengthening. Remember to perform the exercise with control, focusing on maintaining proper form and alignment throughout.

Wall Supported Knee Lifts with Twist

Wall Supported Knee Lifts with Twist is an excellent exercise for enhancing core strength, improving balance, and increasing flexibility. This exercise combines a knee lift with a rotational twist, targeting the obliques, hip flexors, and abdominal muscles. The wall support adds stability, making it accessible for a wide range of fitness levels.

Instructions for Wall Supported Knee Lifts with Twist

1. Starting Position: Stand sideways next to a wall with one hand resting on the wall for support.

2. Movement: Lift the knee closest to the wall towards your chest. Simultaneously, twist your upper body towards the raised knee. Extend your free hand towards the raised knee to deepen the twist.

3. Return: Slowly lower your leg and untwist your upper body to return to the starting position.

4. Breathing: Inhale as you lift your knee and exhale as you twist.

5. Posture: Keep your standing leg slightly bent at the knee. Maintain an upright posture throughout the exercise.

Number of Sets and Repetitions

- ☐ - Beginners: Start with 2 sets of 8 to 10 repetitions on each side. Focus on controlled movements and maintaining balance.
- ☐ - Intermediate: Perform 3 sets of 10 to 12 repetitions per side.
- ☐ - Advanced: Increase the challenge by holding the twist for a few seconds or adding more sets.

Wall Supported Knee Lifts with Twist is a versatile exercise for developing core strength and improving balance. It can be incorporated into a fitness routine focused on core conditioning or used as a standalone exercise for enhancing stability and flexibility.

Remember to perform the exercise with control, focusing on engaging your core muscles and maintaining proper form throughout.

WORKOUT PLAN(28-DAYS CHALLENGE)

28-Day Wall Pilates Challenge: Morning and Evening Routines

Each session should be adjusted to your comfort level. Gradually increase intensity or repetitions as you progress.

Week 1: Foundations

- Day 1
  - Morning: Wall Supported Knee Lifts with Twist (10 reps each side)
  - Evening: Wall-Assisted Lateral Lunges (10 reps each side)
- Day 2
  - Morning: Wall Supported Hip Circles with Arms (8 circles each direction)
  - Evening: Standing Wall Figure Eights with Arms (8 reps each side)
- Day 3

- Morning: Wall-Assisted Bird Dog with Arms (10 reps each side)
- Evening: Wall-Assisted T-spine Rotation (10 reps each side)
- Day 4
- Morning: Wall Balance on One Leg (30 seconds each leg)
- Evening: Wall-Assisted Squat to Toe Touch (10 reps each side)
- Day 5
- Morning: Wall Angel Wings (10 reps)
- Evening: Wall-Assisted Single Leg Deadlift (8 reps each leg)
- Day 6
- Morning: Wall Supported Chair Pose (Hold for 30 seconds)
- Evening: Wall Balance on One Leg with Twist (10 reps each side)
- Day 7
- Morning: Wall Supported Triangle Pose (Hold for 30 seconds each side)
- Evening: Wall Supported Warrior Pose (Hold for 30 seconds each side)

Week 2 - Building Strength and Flexibility

Day 8
- Morning: Wall-Assisted Hamstring Stretch
 (12 reps each side)
- Evening: Wall Supported Hip Circles with Arms
(10 circles each direction)

Day 9
- Morning: Standing Wall Calf Stretch
(10 reps each side)
- Evening: Wall-Assisted Squat to Toe Touch (12
reps each side)

Day 10
- Morning: Wall-Assisted Chest Stretch
(Hold for 40 seconds each leg)
- Evening: Wall-Assisted Single Leg Deadlift (10
reps each leg)

Day 11
- Morning: Wall Angel Wings (12 reps)
- Evening: Wall-Assisted Bird Dog with Arms (12
reps each side)

Day 12
- Morning:Wall-Assisted Quadriceps Stretch
(Hold for 40 seconds)
- Evening: Wall-Supported Side Stretch
(12 reps each side)

Day 13
- Morning: Wall Supported Triangle Pose (Hold for
40 seconds each side)
- Evening: Wall-Assisted Triceps Stretch
 (12 reps each side)

Day 14
- Morning: Wall Supported Forward Bend
 (Hold for 40 seconds each side)
- Evening: Wall-Assisted Spinal Twist
(12 reps)

In this second week, continue to emphasize the
importance of form while gradually increasing the
intensity and duration of each exercise. This week's
focus is on building strength and enhancing
flexibility, creating a solid foundation for more
advanced Wall Pilates exercises. Remember to stay

consistent with your practice and mindful of your body's responses.

Week 3 - Improving Balance and Stability

Day 15
- Morning: Wall Plank
 (Hold for 45 seconds)
- Evening: Wall-Assisted T-spine Rotation (15 reps each side)

Day 16
- Morning: Standing Wall Calf Raises
(12 reps each side)
- Evening: Wall Supported Chair Pose
(Hold 50 seconds)

Day 17
- Morning: Wall Heel-to-Toe Stand
 (15 reps each side)
- Evening: Wall-Assisted Squat to Toe Touch (15 reps each side)

Day 18
- Morning: Wall Supported Warrior Pose (Hold for 45 seconds each side)
- Evening: Wall Supported Triangle Pose (Hold for 45 seconds each side)

Day 19
- Morning: Wall Supported Chair Pose (Hold for 45 seconds)
- Evening: Wall Tree Pose
 (50 seconds hold)

Day 20
- Morning: Wall-Assisted Lateral Lunges (15 reps each side)
- Evening: Wall-Assisted Single Leg Deadlift (12 reps each leg)

Day 21
- Morning: Wall Pelvic Tilts
 (15 reps)
- Evening: Wall Supported Knee Lifts with Twist (15 reps each side)

In week 3, the focus is on enhancing balance and stability. The exercises are designed to challenge your equilibrium and core strength, contributing to a more stable and controlled Pilates practice. As always, adjust the intensity to your comfort level and focus on maintaining proper form throughout each movement.

Week 4 - Focusing on Mobility

Day 22
- Morning: Wall-Assisted Bird Dog with Arms (16 reps each side)
- Evening: Wall Balance on One Leg
 (Hold for 50 seconds)

Day 23
- Morning: Wall-Assisted Squat to Toe Touch
 (Hold for 50 seconds each side)
- Evening: Wall Supported Hip Circles with Arms
(14 circles each direction)

Day 24

- Morning: Wall Balance on One Leg (Hold for 50 seconds each leg)
- Evening: Wall-Assisted Squat to Toe Touch (16 reps each side)

Day 25
- Morning: Wall-Assisted Single Leg Lifts
 (Hold for 50 seconds each side)
- Evening: Standing Wall Figure Eights with Arms (14 reps each side)

Day 26
- Morning: Wall-Assisted Single Leg Deadlift (14 reps each leg)
- Evening: Wall-Assisted T-spine Rotation (16 reps each side)

Day 27
- Morning: Wall Supported Knee Lifts with Twist (16 reps each side)
- Evening: Wall Angel Wings (16 reps)

Day 28
- Morning: Wall Balance on One Leg with Twist (16 reps each side)

- Evening: Wall-Assisted Lateral Lunges (16 reps each side)

In this final week of the challenge, the focus shifts to enhancing mobility. The exercises are specifically chosen to improve the range of motion in your joints, flexibility in your muscles, and overall fluidity of movement. As you approach the end of this challenge, reflect on your progress and how each exercise has contributed to your increased mobility. Continue to listen to your body and adjust the exercises to suit your evolving capabilities.

There will be extra workouts guide for you to choose the exercises suitable for you.

WALL PILATES WEEKLY CHALLENGE

WEEKLY MOTIVATION: "THE ONLY WAY TO ACHIEVE THE IMPOSSIBLE IS TO BELIEVE IT IS POSSIBLE." - CHARLES KINGSLEIGH

	MORNING	AFTERNOON	EVENING
MON			
TUES			
WED			
THURS			
FRI			
SAT			

NOTE ON NEW WEEKLY DISCOVERIES

WALL PILATES WEEKLY CHALLENGE

WEEKLY MOTIVATION: "DO NOT COUNT THE DAYS; MAKE THE DAYS COUNT." - MUHAMMAD ALI.

	MORNING	AFTERNOON	EVENING
MON			
TUES			
WED			
THURS			
FRI			
SAT			

NOTE ON NEW WEEKLY DISCOVERIES

WALL PILATES WEEKLY CHALLENGE

WEEKLY MOTIVATION: "STRENGTH DOES NOT COME FROM PHYSICAL CAPACITY. IT COMES FROM AN INDOMITABLE WILL." - MAHATMA GANDHI

	MORNING	AFTERNOON	EVENING
MON			
TUES			
WED			
THURS			
FRI			
SAT			

NOTE ON NEW WEEKLY DISCOVERIES

WORKOUT SUITABLE RECIPES AND MEAL PLANNER

The efficacy of your Wall Pilates routine is significantly influenced by your dietary choices. The right meal plan plays a pivotal role in determining your energy levels, workout performance, recovery rate, and overall health benefits gained from Wall Pilates.

1. Energy Supply: Pre-workout meals, rich in complex carbohydrates and proteins, provide a steady source of energy, essential for the sustained physical activity of Wall Pilates. These nutrients ensure that you have enough stamina to perform each movement with precision and effectiveness.

2. Muscle Health: Post-workout meals, particularly those high in protein, are crucial for muscle repair and growth. Wall Pilates engages various muscle

groups; adequate protein intake aids in healing and strengthening these muscles, leading to improved performance and reduced risk of injury.

3. Flexibility and Mobility: Foods high in antioxidants and healthy fats, such as omega-3 fatty acids, contribute to joint health and flexibility. Since Wall Pilates involves a range of motions and stretches, maintaining joint health is essential for achieving the full range of movement required.

4. Overall Well-being: Consistent intake of nutrient-dense foods enhances your overall physical health, which in turn impacts your ability to perform Pilates exercises. Nutritional support is crucial for maintaining balance, coordination, and focus - all key elements in executing Wall Pilates effectively.

5. Mental Clarity and Focus: A balanced diet influences cognitive function and mood. Wall Pilates not only demands physical effort but also requires mental engagement. Foods rich in vitamins, minerals, and healthy fats support brain health, ensuring better concentration and a more mindful practice.

In conclusion, integrating a well-balanced meal plan with your Wall Pilates routine is not just about enhancing physical performance; it's about fostering an environment where both body and mind can thrive, leading to a more effective, enjoyable, and beneficial workout experience.

15 Healthy Recipes to Complement Your Wall Pilates Routine

1. Morning Kick-Starter Smoothie
   - Ingredients: Spinach, banana, Greek yogurt, almond milk, honey.
   - Benefit: Provides energy for morning Wall Pilates sessions.

2. Quinoa and Black Bean Salad
   - Ingredients: Quinoa, black beans, cherry tomatoes, avocado, lime juice.
   - Benefit: Great post-workout meal for muscle recovery.

3. Grilled Chicken with Steamed Vegetables
   - Ingredients: Chicken breast, broccoli, carrots, olive oil, herbs.

- Benefit: Lean protein and veggies support muscle repair after Pilates.

4. Avocado Toast with Poached Egg
   - Ingredients: Whole grain bread, avocado, egg, chili flakes.
   - Benefit: Ideal for a pre-workout meal, offering healthy fats and protein.

5. Almond Butter and Banana Smoothie
   - Ingredients: Almond butter, banana, oat milk, cinnamon.
   - Benefit: Quick energy boost before your Pilates session.

6. Greek Yogurt with Berries and Nuts
   - Ingredients: Greek yogurt, mixed berries, almonds, honey.
   - Benefit: Perfect for post-workout recovery with protein and antioxidants.

7. Baked Salmon with Asparagus
   - Ingredients: Salmon fillet, asparagus, lemon, dill.
   - Benefit: Omega-3 fatty acids in salmon enhance joint health.

8. Whole Grain Pasta with Spinach and Pesto
   - Ingredients: Whole grain pasta, spinach, pesto sauce, pine nuts.
   - Benefit: Balanced meal for sustained energy, good for evening Pilates.

9. Tofu Stir-Fry with Brown Rice
   - Ingredients: Tofu, mixed vegetables, brown rice, soy sauce.
   - Benefit: Plant-based protein and fiber-rich meal for muscle building.

10. Kale and Avocado Salad
    - Ingredients: Kale, avocado, cherry tomatoes, lemon dressing.
    - Benefit: Nutrient-packed salad for overall health and vitality.

11. Sweet Potato and Black Bean Chili
    - Ingredients: Sweet potatoes, black beans, tomatoes, chili spices.
    - Benefit: Hearty and healthy, ideal for replenishing energy stores.

12. Oatmeal with Chia Seeds and Apples

- Ingredients: Rolled oats, chia seeds, apple slices, cinnamon.
- Benefit: Provides a slow-release energy, perfect for morning routines.

13. Lentil Soup with Spinach
- Ingredients: Lentils, spinach, carrots, onions, vegetable broth.
- Benefit: Nutrient-rich soup that's great for post-exercise nourishment.

14. Roasted Beet and Goat Cheese Salad
- Ingredients: Roasted beets, goat cheese, walnuts, arugula, balsamic vinaigrette.
- Benefit: Offers vitamins and minerals to support overall fitness.

15. Protein Power Balls
- Ingredients: Oats, peanut butter, honey, flax seeds, protein powder.
- Benefit: Quick snack for an energy boost before or after Pilates.

Using These Recipes with Your Wall Pilates Routine

- Pre-Workout Meals: Choose meals that are light yet energizing, like smoothies or oatmeal, about 30-60 minutes before your Wall Pilates session to fuel your workout.

- Post-Workout Meals: Opt for protein-rich recipes, like grilled chicken or tofu stir-fry, post-workout to aid in muscle recovery and repair.

- Throughout the Day: Maintain balanced nutrition with meals like salads, whole grain pasta, and soups to support overall health and complement your Pilates routine.

Remember, hydration is key, so drink plenty of water before, during, and after your workouts. These recipes, combined with a consistent Wall Pilates routine, will help maximize your health benefits and enhance your overall fitness journey.

14-days Meal Plan for Wall Pilates Routine

Note: Adjust portion sizes according to individual caloric needs.

Week 1:

- Day 1
  - Pre-Workout: Almond Butter and Banana Smoothie
  - Post-Workout: Grilled Chicken with Steamed Vegetables

- Day 2
  - Pre-Workout: Greek Yogurt with Berries and Nuts
  - Post-Workout: Quinoa and Black Bean Salad

- Day 3
  - Pre-Workout: Oatmeal with Chia Seeds and Apples
  - Post-Workout: Baked Salmon with Asparagus

- Day 4

- Pre-Workout: Morning Kick-Starter Smoothie
- Post-Workout: Tofu Stir-Fry with Brown Rice

- Day 5
  - Pre-Workout: Avocado Toast with Poached Egg
  - Post-Workout: Lentil Soup with Spinach

- Day 6
  - Pre-Workout: Protein Power Balls
  - Post-Workout: Whole Grain Pasta with Spinach and Pesto

- Day 7
  - Pre-Workout: Greek Yogurt with Berries and Nuts
  - Post-Workout: Sweet Potato and Black Bean Chili

Week 2:

- Day 8
  - Pre-Workout: Almond Butter and Banana Smoothie
  - Post-Workout: Kale and Avocado Salad

- Day 9

- Pre-Workout: Oatmeal with Chia Seeds and Apples
- Post-Workout: Grilled Chicken with Steamed Vegetables

- Day 10
  - Pre-Workout: Morning Kick-Starter Smoothie
  - Post-Workout: Baked Salmon with Asparagus

- Day 11
  - Pre-Workout: Avocado Toast with Poached Egg
  - Post-Workout: Tofu Stir-Fry with Brown Rice

- Day 12
  - Pre-Workout: Greek Yogurt with Berries and Nuts
  - Post-Workout: Quinoa and Black Bean Salad

- Day 13
  - Pre-Workout: Protein Power Balls
  - Post-Workout: Lentil Soup with Spinach

- Day 14
  - Pre-Workout: Oatmeal with Chia Seeds and Apples

- Post-Workout: Roasted Beet and Goat Cheese Salad

This meal plan is designed to provide balanced nutrition to support your Wall Pilates routine, focusing on energizing pre-workout meals and nourishing post-workout meals for recovery and strength.

CONCLUSION

As we reach the conclusion of this journey through "Wall Pilates Workouts for Men," it's important to reflect on the key lessons and benefits we've discovered. This book has been a guide to enhancing your physical well-being, focusing on strength, flexibility, balance, and coordination, all through the innovative use of wall-assisted exercises.

The exercises presented here are more than just a series of movements; they are part of a holistic approach to health and fitness, especially tailored for men over 40. The wall, an often overlooked piece of 'equipment', has shown its versatility in providing support, stability, and resistance, making Pilates more accessible and effective.

Remember, the journey to better health is ongoing. Consistency and dedication are key. Incorporating these exercises into your routine can lead to significant improvements in posture, core strength, and overall physical health. Whether you're a seasoned athlete or just beginning your fitness journey, these wall-assisted exercises can be adapted to your level and needs.

As you continue to practice and grow stronger, allow yourself to experiment and explore variations of these exercises. Listen to your body, understand its limits, and gradually push those boundaries to achieve greater flexibility and strength.

Above all, let this book be a reminder that age is not a barrier to fitness and well-being. With the right approach, guidance, and determination, maintaining and improving your physical health is always within reach. Keep challenging yourself, stay motivated, and enjoy the journey towards a healthier, stronger you.

Thank you for reading

Thank you so much for choosing and reading my book! Your support means the world to me. If you enjoyed your journey through the pages, I would be incredibly grateful if you could take a moment to leave a positive feedback on Amazon. Your feedback not only helps me grow as an author but also assists fellow readers in discovering this book. Thank you once again for being an amazing part of my writing journey!